WHAT DOCTORS ARE SAYING ABOUT DR. KOTLUS

"As the President-Elect of the American Academy of Cosmetic Surgery, I have been afforded the opportunity to get to know colleagues across the country and abroad. After awhile, it becomes easily apparent who some of the leaders in cosmetic surgery will be. Dr. Kotlus is one of these surgeons who stands out above most of the crowd. He is one few surgeons who has devoted an extra year of training beyond his residency to complete a cosmetic surgery fellowship. Dr. Kotlus is a very active member of the AACS, lecturing at national meetings and serving on committees. His personality, training and natural gifts have given him the ability to produce a wonderful basic guide for the average patient seeking cosmetic surgery. I applaud his efforts to create something for our cosmetic surgery patients that is educational and easy to understand."

★ Angelo Cuzalina, MD
President Elect of the American Academy of Cosmetic Surgery

"Brett Kotlus is an authority in the field of cosmetic surgery. More than that he is a promoter of public safety and education and is a reliable resource for practitioners in the field of cosmetic surgery as well as those contemplating having cosmetic surgery performed for their own needs. I am proud to have him as a friend and colleague."

★ Edward B. Lack MD
Past President, American Academy of Cosmetic Surgery

"Dr. Kotlus is a very qualified cosmetic surgeon and is well versed and trained in both facial and body cosmetic surgery. He is well known to his peers as a surgeon, author and researcher and always seems to be on the cutting edge of contemporary cosmetic surgery. Dr. Kotlus has the unique ability to look at complex situations and reduce them to easily understood basics. This ability makes Brett the perfect author for a textbook that is designed to simplify and elucidate many of the complex questions and concerns about cosmetic surgery.

Unfortunately, much cosmetic surgery information is warped by myth, legend, competitive concerns among surgeons. The media and industry often put forth unreliable information about cosmetic surgery and Dr. Kotlus has set out to answer the important questions and provide accurate material to arm the prospective cosmetic surgery patient with the facts. For the price of a lunch, this book could save patients thousands of dollars of unnecessary or unproven surgery as well as the frustration of trying to figure out fact from fiction."

★ **Joe Niamtu, III DMD**
Cosmetic Facial Surgeon

"Dr. Brett Kotlus is a highly qualified cosmetic surgeon. His book, Boost Your Beauty, offers the reader clear advice on cosmetic surgery in language that is clear and easy to understand. This resource will help anyone considering cosmetic surgery by offering plain talk on the risks and benefits of the popular cosmetic surgeries. The need for this type of clear thinking from a well-trained surgeon is all the more important to cut through the confusing array of misinformation on the Internet. Much of this misinformation is written or republished by non-surgeons who pass on information with no direct working knowledge except perhaps a single personal experience with a plastic surgeon. Readers will benefit from the detailed descriptions of who should and should not have surgery, and what to expect after surgery. The reader will also find solid information about individual types of surgery free from the biases of more commercial resources found on the Internet.

Dr. Kotlus is to be congratulated for this excellent contribution."

★ **Kenneth D. Steinsapir, M.D.**
Associate Clinical Professor, Jules Stein Eye Institute
The David Geffen School of Medicine at UCLA

WHAT PATIENTS ARE SAYING ABOUT DR. KOTLUS

"I have had the most wonderful experience so far at Allure. I've been to about 5 different treatments centers for my veins and I haven't had a good experience until Allure. At Allure, I finally feel comfortable and encouraged...I've always felt so embarrassed. I have been telling everyone what a great experience I am having and will definitely recommend." ★ **Jena**

"[My breast augmentation] looks so natural. I got saline implants, and Dr. Kotlus never tried to talk me into the more expensive silicone. He went through my belly button so I wouldn't have any scars. I love them totally. When I've shown my girlfriends, and they've known other gals that have done it, they say they're the most natural-looking pair they have ever seen. He did such a great job...he was so calm and so professional and realistic. Seeing my results now, I would have it done sooner. I feel sexier than I ever have...and I'm 46!" ★ **Julia**

"Everyone was very attentive, friendly and seemed happy that I was there. I also liked that Dr. Kotlus is so professional and knowledgeable. The office was very busy but he acted like he had all the time in the world for me and answered all of my questions." ★ **Melissa**

"Before the procedure, in order to look directly ahead, I would have to elevate my head. Because of the puffiness my eyelids looked half closed. Now after the surgery, everybody's really noticed the fact that my eyes really open up. Now people notice my facial expressions, no doubt about it. It's a hundred and ten percent improvement!" ★ **Gene**

"When I went in for my first procedure, I was so embarrassed about my legs I cried. They were really unsightly. All these green veins; it's not pretty. The staff made me feel so comfortable. They're wonderful, and they share their own stories from different procedures. They were so open that you leave there hugging people. My daughter came with me to every procedure. They encouraged her questions. They let her come in to the room. They explained everything – every step of the way...I can't say enough about them and their procedures and their staff. I can't recommend them enough!" ★ **Renata**

"I had a lot of excess skin underneath my face and chin, and I just wasn't happy with the way I looked. Anytime someone would be taking pictures, I'd always shy away from the camera...The thing that really pushed me to [have a neck lift] was my daughter's wedding. My daughter kept saying, 'I want you in the wedding pictures.'...My daughter got married a month after my procedure and people just thought I looked really good- nobody knew what I had done...People were saying, 'Did you lose weight? Something looks different.' It was pretty dramatic- they just thought I looked really young." ★ **Grace**

"[The tummy tuck] only took a few hours and immediately you could see the results...The next day my stomach was completely flat...Three weeks later, it was my cousin's wedding, and I did the alligator on the floor with my sisters. I was pretty good!" ★ **Katie**

"Dr. Kotlus, thank you SO much! I love the way my neck looks. You have done a fantastic job! My husband was also very impressed with you and said that you are a man of integrity. You are the best! Thank you!" ★ **Marty**

ABOUT THE AUTHOR

Brett Kotlus, M.D., M.S is a cosmetic and oculofacial plastic surgeon, having completed two accredited fellowships in oculofacial plastic and cosmetic surgery. A respected publisher of numerous scientific articles, he has presented his research at national scientific conferences. Dr. Kotlus is also a national instructor in facelift and rhinoplasty surgery. Recently, Dr. Kotlus' teaching have taken him to Mongolia on a medical mission to instruct local doctors. In 2007, he was the first recipient of two Cosmetic Surgery Foundation research grants.

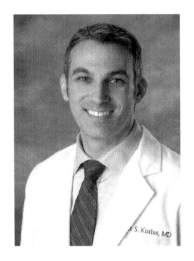

Dr. Kotlus received his medical degree from the Sackler School of Medicine at Tel Aviv University. While completing his residency in Ophthalmology at the North Shore-Long Island Jewish Health System of the Albert Einstein College of Medicine in New York, he held the prestigious position of Chief Resident. He received his Master's degree in Genetics at the Pennsylvania State University.

Board Certifications:

★ American Board of Cosmetic Surgery - Diplomate

★ American Board of Ophthalmology - Diplomate

Professional Affiliations:

★ Michigan Society of Cosmetic Surgery - Founder

★ American Academy of Cosmetic Surgery - Fellow

★ American Society of Ophthalmic Plastic and Reconstructive Surgery - Fellow

★ American Academy of Ophthalmology - Fellow

★ Phi Beta Kappa - Member

ALSO BY BRETT KOTLUS

"Functional and Cosmetic Surgery Intersect in a Positive Way"

★ Ocular Surgery News

"Facelift Enhancement with the Wire Scalpel"

★ Cosmetic Surgery Times

"Folds and Creases"

with Dryden, R.M., ★ Plastic Reconstructive Surgery

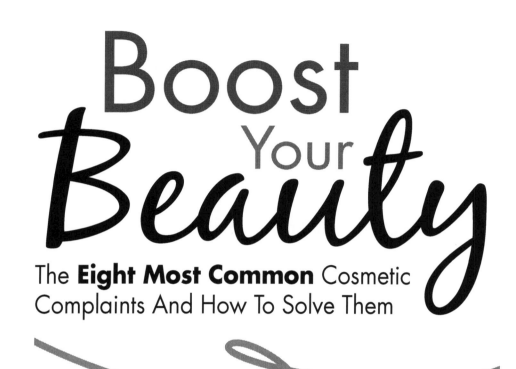

Boost Your Beauty

The **Eight Most Common** Cosmetic Complaints And How To Solve Them

BRETT KOTLUS, M.D.

COSMETIC AND OCULOFACIAL PLASTIC SURGEON

BOOST YOUR BEAUTY
Eight of the Most Common Cosmetic Complaints And How To Solve Them

Dr. Brett Kotlus

Allure Medical Spa
8180 26 Mile Road, Suite 300
Shelby Township, MI 48316
800-577-2570

Find us on the worldwide web at *http://www.alluremedicalspa.com*

To report errors, please send a note to *info@alluremedicalspa.com*

Book design by Leigh Ference-Kaemmer • www.ferencekaemmerdesign.com

Boost Your Beauty

Contents ★

Preface ★

The decision to undergo cosmetic surgery is never an easy one. There are several key issues to consider in your journey. You probably have fear and unanswered questions, as well as conflicting information. I value your desire of becoming a better you and recognize that getting started is most of the work. I am here to help you, to answer your questions, and to guide you through this decision. Mostly, I am here to help you achieve your goals in whatever way I can.

It is my role to educate you about the changes that are possible with cosmetic surgery, and the safest and most sensible way to carry out these changes. The popularity of cosmetic surgery continues to increase and covers a broad demographic of females as well as males. It is being performed throughout the world on a daily basis. All of your needs must be considered individually because there is no single answer that applies to everyone.

Cosmetic surgery is a serious matter; I do not take it lightly and neither should you. Cosmetic surgery alters your appearance. It involves risks and it can be costly. I think it is important for you to have a clear understanding of what is involved before proceeding with any surgery. Cosmetic surgery is only appropriate when it is done by the right doctor, in the right place, at the right time, and for the right reasons.

My intention in writing this book is to help men and women navigate their journey through plastic surgery. As a surgeon, my mission is to erase the confusion and answer all of the questions you may have about cosmetic surgery. I am excited to enlighten you about the positive benefits cosmetic surgery holds for you and your body, and I want to diminish any trepidation you are experiencing in making your decision. I wish to leave a lasting impression on your mind and in your heart that I care deeply for every one of my patients.

I hope you use this book as a road map through the world of cosmetic surgery. I wish you the best in achieving your goals.

Brett Kotlus, M.D.

Introduction ★

A couple of decades ago, there was a much stronger stigma associated with having cosmetic surgery. Today, however, more than 11 million cosmetic procedures are performed every single year. About 60% of Americans say they approve of cosmetic surgery and nearly 80% say they would not be embarrassed if people outside of their immediate family learned about their cosmetic procedure.

Modern techniques have also made cosmetic surgery much more accessible and effective than it once was, but how do you know if a cosmetic procedure is right for you?

Are you ready for cosmetic surgery?

When deciding whether or not to undergo cosmetic surgery, there is much more to consider than just whether you are dissatisfied with your appearance. You must look at your lifestyle, finances, and most importantly, the roots of your desire to change how you look. The first chapter of this book delves in to this question and encourages you evaluate yourself carefully to be sure that you are a good candidate for cosmetic surgery.

The goal of this book is to help educate you about common cosmetic surgical procedures and encourage you to weigh your alternatives. Always remember that cosmetic surgery is a big decision. Consider your options seriously and carefully.

Why have cosmetic surgery?

People have many reasons for getting cosmetic procedures done. I see people on both sides of the spectrum in my practice. They may come in for the right reasons or the wrong reasons. Everyone has a unique reason or set of reasons for having cosmetic surgery. Examples of reasons I have heard over the years include:

★ A patient wants to improve a "bothersome" area of their body that has been upsetting them for a long time.

★ A patient wants to correct an anatomic issue with their body.

★ A patient wants to fix a genetic problem with their body.

★ A patient wants to enhance a part of their body that they like but would like to "shine through" a little more.

My practice is a busy one, and I perform hundreds of procedures each month. Each day I consult with prospective patients (including many who have never had a cosmetic procedure). In the initial consultation, I make it a point to probe the real motivations behind the decision to have cosmetic surgery. Part of my job is to help determine whether or not they have the right motivation.

For example, I recently saw a female patient who was in good physical shape and had what she referred to as "saddle bags," which were pockets of fat on part of the outer part of her legs. She said that she had always had them, as did her mother. She told me that no matter what amount of exercise she did, and however much weight she lost (or gained), she always had that feature, and it bothered her when she wears a bathing suit. I would refer to her as a very good candidate.

Why not to have cosmetic surgery

Often I view my role as the "voice of reason" for many patients who are considering surgery. For some patients who think that cosmetic surgery is the answer to their problem, I am often the bearer of "bad news." Let me discuss a few instances where I question the motivation to have cosmetic surgery:

★ A patient who incorrectly thinks that cosmetic surgery is going to make their life better overall.

★ A patient incorrectly thinks that cosmetic surgery is going to make someone like them.

★ A patient who unfortunately had someone tell them they need cosmetic surgery.

★ A patient who is under financial hardship should consider if cosmetic surgery is truly a priority.

Ultimately, you are the only person who will know if you are having a procedure done for the right reason. Be honest with yourself.

I'll give you an example of a not-so-good candidate. I often see a prospective patient who is extremely overweight, and is looking toward cosmetic surgery to help remove excess weight. The patient wanted had a hard time losing weight and was interested in liposuction. In this situation, cosmetic surgery would not be the appropriate choice. I stress that their lifestyle needs to be in order first - both diet and exercise - before they can move forward to something cosmetic.

Realistic Expectations

Having realistic expectations is really what determines whether or not someone will be in the right frame of mind before they undergo a procedure.

The patient and the doctor must be speaking in the same terms, and on the same page. Your doctor and you should be in complete agreement on the following questions:

★ What are the goals of the cosmetic procedure?

★ What are the realistic outcomes of the procedure I'm considering?

★ What does the procedure aiming to treat specifically? What won't it treat?

★ What are the (minor and major) risks are in the procedure?

Unrealistic Expectations

Let me give you a common example of an unrealistic expectation. Often people come to see me hoping they can "turn back the clock" with a procedure such as a face lift. Some patients are pleasantly surprised to find out they can often turn back the clock five, or even ten years. Those are realistic expectations.

However, if they think a fifty-year-old can look like eighteen again, that would be unrealistic. A smoker thinking they can eliminate twenty years of smoking with a laser treatment would be unrealistic too. There is a limit as to how each procedure will work on a patient, and the patient must know those limits.

Your doctor can help you understand realistic expectations by showing example of before and after photos. Often patients bring in pictures of famous people, and they'll want the nose, chin, or cheeks a famous actor. You can certainly use these as a guidepost, but you need to be careful. Your doctor will be able to guide expectations in situations like these, because people in magazines are often airbrushed. There's sort of a pop culture dialogue that says everyone should be "perfect," but often that "perfection" is unrealistic. And remember, your features are different than someone else's. After any procedure, you will still be you.

Are you a good candidate for cosmetic surgery?

When determining if you are a good candidate for a cosmetic procedure, you should consider the physical and emotional (or psychological) perspective. You may be a good candidates from a physical perspective, but perhaps you are not be a good candidate from an emotional or psychological perspective. There are many considerations you must have before moving forward.

The first step involves looking in the mirror. Is there something about your appearance that bothers you when you look in the mirror? Or is it something that bothers you because someone else said something about "it"? It is critically important that the decision to have a cosmetic procedure comes internally.

This is something I always stress during the first meeting with a patient. Cosmetic surgery is something that someone does for themselves, and to feel better about themselves. You should absolutely not do it for anyone else. It's something you do when you want your external features to project the person you feel you are the inside.

Overall Health

Patients need to prioritize overall well being when considering any kind of elective surgery. If your health isn't at an optimal level, don't consider elective surgery - even minimally invasive surgery. If you have poorly controlled diabetes or hypertension that isn't controlled, then having an elective liposuction procedure would not be a good choice. You simply aren't a good candidate - at that time. Medical conditions take priority in terms of what you should address before you undergo any cosmetic surgery. For an elective procedure for your appearance, it's simply not worth the risk if you are not healthy.

A few other examples. In general, people who are smokers are not always great candidates for invasive cosmetic procedures because smoking interferes with the body's healing process. People who have serious medical conditions - even when they are controlled - often need to have a consultation with their primary care doctor or their specialists whether it is advisable to move forward.

It also may be the case that someone who is not a candidate for one procedure may be a candidate for another. I've had a patient that wasn't an appropriate candidate for a facelift, for example, but was a great candidate for something less invasive - something that did not require anesthesia - such as BOTOX®, fillers, or even laser surfacing. Ultimately, the procedure a patient chooses (and is approved for) has to be tailored to the patient's specific goals, their expectations, and their medical conditions.

Your cosmetic surgeon will tell you which options are really good options for you and which ones shouldn't be considered at certain times. It is sometimes the case that someone who is taking a blood thinner (due to a medical condition) would be able to stop the blood thinner for a period of time to have a filler injection. Changing a medication regimen in this way would be done in conjunction with your primary care doctor or specialist.

Bad Habits

If I could I wave a magic wand, I'd like to have all of my patients to stop smoking. I think everyone knows that smoking is not good for them. However, not everyone always knows that smoking interferes with healing after surgery or even that smoking leaves more wrinkles. It's common for someone to come in for a consultation and feel discouraged when you they are told as long as they continue smoking, they will continue to have lines on their face and that it will be harder to get rid of them. In fact, they will probably progress.

After talking to thousands of patients who smoke, I realize it is difficult to stop bad habits like smoking. It's something that many of patients struggle with. I think it is easy to feel discouraged when you feel you have a liability such as a smoking habit or history of significant sun exposure. It's important to note that these things can be managed, and it is possible for people with a smoking habit to improve their appearance. Sometimes the notion that there is a a cosmetic procedure that may help them down the road might give them motivation to address their habit today.

I don't pretend that it's easy to deal with difficult lifestyle issues. It's easy for me to say you have to stop smoking, but I sympathize with patients who have an addiction or have a habit. I realize that it takes a lot of effort to overcome. It also means that when they do overcome it, the results can be so much more rewarding.

Risks

Everything we do is associated with some risk. The risks associated with cosmetic surgery are real and should certainly be considered when making the decision to undergo a procedure. The chances of having a complication after a cosmetic procedure vary widely. These depend on a number of factors, including some unknown factors. Some of the less invasive procedures tend to have minor risks such as swelling, bruising, and redness. There are more serious risks associated with surgery including bleeding, infection, and scarring. Even the anesthesia required to keep you comfortable during a procedure has risks.

Your doctor will review some of the possible risks with you before a procedure, and you will be asked to sign a consent form stating that you understand the risks. It is impossible to anticipate every potential complication that could arise from a procedure. But there are things you can do to minimize risks, such as smoking cessation and following your doctor's instructions before and after a procedure. You should ask your doctor what will be done in the unfortunate case that you do experience a complication.

Cosmetic surgery versus plastic surgery

People often confuse the terms cosmetic surgery and plastic surgery, but they are not exactly the same. Cosmetic surgery aims to improve the appearance through surgical procedures. Such procedures include liposuction, face lifts, breast enhancements, and modifications of that nature. Plastic surgery is a discipline of medicine that can deal with appearance but also deals with reconstructive aspects of medicine. Reconstructive procedures include treating burns, trauma, rearrangements after cancer surgeries, etc..

So there's an overlap between plastic surgery and cosmetic surgery. Not every plastic surgeon is trained in cosmetic procedures and not every cosmetic surgeon is trained in all plastic procedures. Cosmetic surgeons can come from a variety of medical disciplines which include dermatology, otolaryngology, oculofacial surgery, gynecology, to name a few. In fact, the most common procedures in cosmetic surgery originated from disciplines other than plastic surgery. For example, tumescent liposuction techniques which have increased the safety of the procedure were developed and popularized by a dermatologist. Cosmetic BOTOX® and medical lasers for example, were both pioneered by ophthalmologists.

Credentials of cosmetic surgeons will vary. Many physicians will undergo fellowship training in cosmetic surgery, meaning that they spend an extended period of time learning cosmetic surgical procedures in an accredited program. I spent two years in a cosmetic surgery fellowship after my residency. Some cosmetic surgeons acquire more skills after their formal training. In choosing a doctor, you want to have a procedure done with somebody who would feel comfortable with that particular procedure, meaning they have the experience and training. It is important to look at the quality of the work that they've done before in terms of before and after photos and in speaking to other patients.

The American Board of Cosmetic Surgery (ABCS) is the only board that certifies doctors in surgery of the appearance, specifically. A cosmetic surgeon may have certification from other boards which are members of

American Board of Medical Specialties, or ABMS. So this physician may have a board certification in Ear, Nose, Throat Surgery, or in Dermatology, or Ophthalmology, but then they would have done further training in cosmetic surgery in order to get to that specialized level. In order to be board certified in cosmetic surgery, a physician would have to show proof of training and experience. And then that surgeon will sit for a full day oral and written examination. So after going through that process, and doing it successfully, he or she would be considered to be credentialed by the American Board of Cosmetic Surgery. There is also the American Society of Cosmetic Surgery, which accreditates specific training programs in cosmetic surgery and offers educational resources for surgeons. That being said, I know some excellent surgeons who are not certified by the ABCS and are highly skilled. You are obligated to ask questions and do some rudimentary research to determine if you are choosing the right person.

How much does cosmetic surgery cost?

Cost is an important factor to weigh when considering cosmetic surgery. Before you commit to anything, you should make sure you're working within your means.

Nearly all cosmetic procedures are considered elective, which means that your health insurance company won't foot the bill. A couple of procedures – namely, breast reductions and eyelid lifts – are occasionally covered by insurance when your circumstances could be considered dangerous to your health. These options are discussed in more detail in their respective chapters. For now, it's safest to assume that your cosmetic procedure will need to be paid for out of your own pocket.

The fees for each type of procedure vary widely from doctor to doctor and from state to state. There may also be different options for the procedure that you are interested in that can increase or reduce the cost. Your doctor can help you understand what results each of your options can produce and help you strike a balance between optimal results and any budgetary constraints.

You can and should interview several doctors before settling on someone to perform your cosmetic procedure. Make sure your doctor factors in all costs, including consultation time, anesthesia, post-procedural care items, checkups and, of course, the procedure itself. That way you can be sure there will be no unpleasant surprises when you get the bill.

Which doctor is right for me?

Of course, price should not be the only factor in your choice of doctor. It is critical that you check into a cosmetic surgeon's experience with the specific kind of procedure you require and ask a lot of questions. It's in the best interests of both yourself and your doctor to be an informed, involved patient who understands all aspects of your chosen treatment.

Each chapter comes with a checklist of key points to cover with your doctor, so be sure to bring this book along to your consultation appointments. Write down the answers to your questions so that you can refer to them later, and don't be shy about voicing any other questions that come up during your decision making process.

Also, don't be afraid to ask for at least a few current references. Experienced, qualified surgeons should not hesitate to provide you with contact information for three to five of their previous patients. Make sure the references you receive are people who have undergone a similar procedure to the one you are interested in having done yourself.

Above all, trust your instincts. It's important to have a great rapport with your doctor so that you feel as comfortable as possible before, during, and after your cosmetic procedure. When you find that perfect chemistry with an experienced, approachable surgeon who cares about your concerns and has your best interest in mind, you'll know you've found the right person to help give you the appearance you deserve.

How this book is organized

Each of the most common types of cosmetic procedures has its own chapter in this book. You will find information on:

★ **Sagging eyelids:** Stretched skin around your eyes can make you look older than you are and, in some cases, actually impede your vision. An eyelid lift can easily remove excess skin in your eye area to make your eyes look more youthful and alert.

★ **Tired-looking eyes:** As you age, the areas around your eyes can lose their natural contours and appear sunken and dark, resulting in tired, old-looking eyes. Your cosmetic surgeon has solutions to firm up and add shape back to the area and get rid of dark circles and hollows under your eyes.

★ **Unsightly veins:** Varicose and spider veins are a common complaint. They're unattractive and can even be quite painful. Whether they're on your legs, hands, or anywhere else on your body, your cosmetic surgeon has simple treatments available to reduce or eliminate the appearance of those unwelcome veins.

★ **Facial treatments:** There are a number of treatments available in a variety of price ranges to help minimize any unwanted lines or wrinkles and/or improve your skin's texture. The result is smoother, more radiant, younger looking skin.

★ **Breast concerns:** Many women complain of breasts that are too small, too large, or too droopy. Cosmetic procedures can enhance or reduce the size of your breasts to create a natural look that improves your silhouette. If your breasts are sagging, your cosmetic surgeon can lift them so they look more pert and youthful.

★ **Unwanted fat:** For stubborn fat deposits that seem to stick around despite your best efforts, liposuction or other treatments may be the solution. Your doctor can help you choose the best way to get rid of any pockets of fat and improve the overall shape of your figure

★ **Droopy necks and jaw lines:** Overstretched skin, usually due to aging, can cause the appearance of unattractive "jowls" along your neckline. A cosmetic surgeon has a number of options to tighten up the area so your jaw and neck look more youthful.

★ **Tummy tucks:** This procedure tightens up your abdominal area by removing hanging, excess skin, resulting in a flatter, more attractive tummy. Sometimes your doctor can also remove excess fat and tighten loose muscles during a tummy tuck.

Within each chapter, you will find five main sections. Each of these sections has been written to help you understand the procedure in question and educate you about your options:

★ **What can this procedure do for me?** This leading section opens up every chapter by introducing what may have led you to consider a specific cosmetic procedure as well as an overview of your potential outcomes, both physical and psychological.

★ **What are my options?** This section highlights the main types of treatments available with the cosmetic procedure in question. You'll learn what specific issues can be treated and how.

★ **Will it hurt?** Pain is a natural concern for anyone considering cosmetic surgery. Although most procedures are quite painless, this section will give you the details about what sensations to expect during your actual treatment as well the types of anesthesia that can be involved.

★ **What about after my treatment?** This section discusses your recovery timeline including how long it will take before you're back on your feet and when you can return to work. You'll also learn about post-treatment care routines that may be necessary until you are fully healed.

★ **What am I going to look like when it's all done?** This is likely the biggest question on your mind. In this section, you'll learn about what outcomes you can realistically expect from your procedure. You'll also learn about potential scarring and the permanence of the treatment being discussed.

Chapter 1 ★

Options For Your Eyelids

★ CHAPTER HIGHLIGHTS:

★ Aging and/or genetics can cause eyelid skin to become droopy. An eyelid lift is a simple cosmetic procedure that can correct this by removing excess skin.

★ Upper and lower eyelid procedures both exist; you may be a candidate for one or both.

★ Eyelid lifts are typically performed under local anesthetic and are therefore pain-free, but you can usually request a sedative if you're feeling anxious.

★ You may experience a variety of side effects from your surgery, the most common of which are swelling, bruising, dry eyes, temporary vision changes, and sensitivity to light and wind. Your doctor can give you medications or advice to help alleviate any discomfort you may feel.

★ You may be able to return to work as soon as the day after surgery, although complete recovery can take one to two weeks.

★ Your new, firmer eyelids can take years off your appearance and improve your peripheral vision.

★ There is often a barely visible scar from this procedure. The healed incision usually fades to a thin, white line that is hidden in the natural crease of your eyelid.

★ Fees vary widely and you may be eligible for insurance coverage.

Can an eyelid lift improve my appearance?

As we age – or sometimes just because of an unfortunate combination of genes – the skin around our eyes can begin to look a little droopy. Some of us try to cover it up with makeup or expensive spa treatments, but nothing really does the trick.

You may be well aware of the negative impact sagging eye skin can have on your overall appearance. It can be really discouraging to have a friend or colleague say, "Are you okay? You look a little sad," or "Wow, you look tired today!" or "What's wrong? You seem angry," when you don't feel sad or tired or angry at all.

Even mild cases of sagging eyelids can have another aggravating effect: vision impairment. Because the skin is effectively "falling down" around your eyes, your peripheral vision can be affected and you may even feel like there's a constant shadow just above your line of sight. In some cases the degree of visual impairment is actually a serious danger to your safety.

★ FAST FACT

Eyelid lifts are one of the top three most common cosmetic procedures performed in the U.S. every single year.

Thankfully, these concerns can be easily corrected with an eyelid lift – also known as "blepharoplasty" – that is performed by a cosmetic surgeon. This simple procedure can dramatically improve the appearance of your eyes and give you a new outlook on life – literally.

If your eyelid skin is seriously impeding your vision, you may actually be eligible to have your corrective cosmetic procedure covered by your medical insurance. This is because enough excess drooping is actually considered a visual impairment and therefore may fall within the scope of your medical coverage.

To determine if you're eligible for your insurance company to foot the bill,

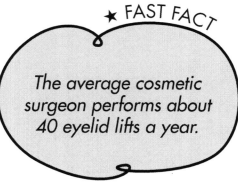

★ FAST FACT

The average cosmetic surgeon performs about 40 eyelid lifts a year.

your surgeon will perform a simple test that involves measuring your peripheral vision twice: once with your skin as it is normally and once with the excess taped up. If the degree of difference is big enough, your insurance company may be willing to pay for your eyelid lift.

Your eyes are the most expressive part of your face; people notice your eyes before they notice any other part of your body. Youthful eyes can express a great deal of energy and happiness. If you've developed sagging skin around your eyes, eyelid surgery may be just the trick to revitalize your appearance so your eyes can express exactly what you want them to.

What are my options?

The two major types of eyelid procedures are upper and lower blepharoplasty, which – you guessed it! – are for your upper and lower eye areas. You may be a candidate for one or both procedures, depending on the location and severity of your sagging eyelid skin.

Upper eyelid lift (upper blepharoplasty)

An upper eyelid lift involves making a tiny incision between your eyebrow and eyelid to remove extra tissue. A skilled surgeon will place the incision in the natural crease of your eyelid, just below your brow bone.

During your procedure, the doctor will essentially use the incision to re-sculpt your eyelid. Extra skin will be cut away and your remaining skin will be pulled up and sutured into place. The goal of the procedure is to eliminate excess skin so you'll be able to see the outside world, free and unencumbered.

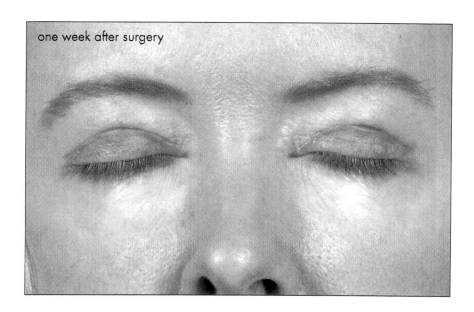

one week after surgery

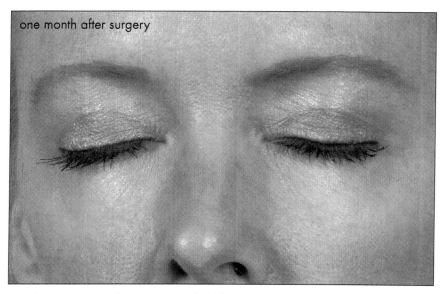

one month after surgery

Healing process after upper eyelid lift at one week after surgery (left) and one month after surgery (right). At one month, the scar is barely visible in the eyelid crease.

Lower eyelid lift (lower blepharoplasty)

Lower blepharoplasty, on the other hand, can take care of unsightly bags under your eyes that make you look tired and grumpy. Like upper blepharoplasty, a small incision is made to remove any excess tissue and firm up the area beneath your eye. Often, this incision is made on the inside of the eyelid, so there is no visible scar to the outside world.

Many surgeons used to remove a lot of fat from the lower eyelids of patients having a lower eyelid lift. These days, it is understood that not everyone requires fat removal. In some cases, patients are hollow under their eyes, creating shadows that can only be improved by actually restoring volume by adding fat or filler. If your lower eyelids need work, a customized approach is necessary to address the specific issues seen by your doctor. A cookie-cutter is simply not the answer.

Important information about blepharoplasty

Both procedures aim to correct sagging eyelids and hollowness. The skin around your eye is the thinnest on your body, which means it is very prone to stretching over time. Your skin does have a remarkable elastic quality, but over the years the connective tissue tends to weaken, which causes skin to lose its ability to rebound. After a certain point, your stretching skin can really only be corrected surgically.

Even an area as small as your eye can have excess muscle and bulging fat, which is why many procedures also involve the removal of these types of tissues. Removal of fat and/or muscle is normal during eyelid surgery

★ FAST FACT

About 250,000 people get eyelid surgery every year in North America.

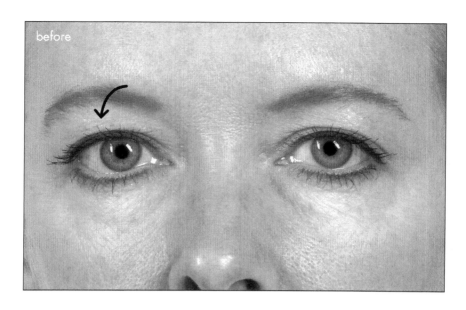

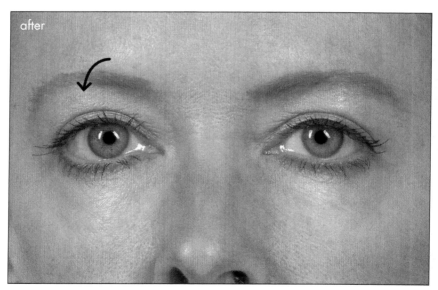

This patient had an upper eyelid lift to correct
her slightly loose upper eyelid skin.

and can go a long way in creating the alert, youthful eyes you're after.

Whichever type of eyelid surgery you have, you will have the opportunity to discuss the look you would like to create during a consultation.

Male and female patients often have different goals in mind for their eyelid surgery. Women tend to like a taut, smooth area that gives them younger-looking eyes and a natural place to apply their makeup. On the other hand, men often prefer a more "relaxed" look. They want their eyes to look mature and sophisticated, but not too old or too young. Again, be clear with your doctor about what your preferences are; your doctor can explain how a realistic outcome might look.

Will my eyelid lift hurt?

Although you will likely be awake during your eyelid lift, most people find the procedure to be extremely tolerable. Eyelid procedures are done under local anesthesia, which means your eye area will be numbed for the length of the surgery to avoid any sensation of pain. Local anesthesia also carries far fewer risks than general anesthesia, but be sure to speak with your doctor about any questions you have regarding anesthesia.

You can expect to feel a tiny amount of pressure or tugging as your doctor performs your eyelid lift. These feelings are completely normal and usually not uncomfortable, but you may be able to request an anti-anxiety medication if you're really nervous about your procedure.

What about after my eyelid lift?

Your eyes will require a certain degree of care after your eyelid lift. Because there has been an incision, you can expect a small amount of

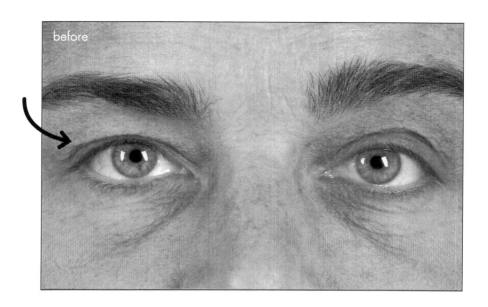

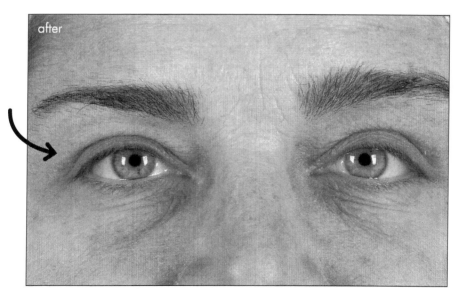

This patient was bothered by the asymmetry between her eyelids. She had an upper eyelid lift on both sides to improve loose skin and make eyelids appear more symmetrical.

swelling, discomfort, and perhaps some minor bruising. You may also temporarily experience dry eyes and irritation. All of these symptoms can last between one and two weeks. Most serious complications are rare.

In the meantime, you can control all of these symptoms with cold compresses, ointment and/or eye drops, and over-the-counter pain medication. Your doctor will prescribe the medications you need and give you detailed post-operative instructions for how to care for your eyes and minimize discomfort while they are healing.

You will be able to go back to work as soon as you are comfortable doing so. If you don't mind your coworkers seeing your bruising from the procedure, you can return to the office as early as the day following your surgery. Driving is also usually okay after your first twenty-four hours have elapsed post-surgery, but you should avoid exercise for about two weeks.

While your eyes are recovering from the procedure, you must be very diligent about sun protection. That means wearing quality sunglasses every time you are in the sun. Remember, the skin around your eyes is very thin and delicate; you'll need to protect it until it's fully healed.

There are a number of procedures that can be combined with eyelid lifts to create a better, longer lasting, more pleasing result. These include BOTOX® treatments to relax frown lines around the eyes, laser resurfacing to help tighten loose skin, or filler and fat injections to plump up hollow areas. Your doctor will suggest some options if you are a candidate for any of these enhancements.

In many cases, BOTOX®, fillers, and lasers can help to maintain the results you have achieved with blepharoplasty;

★ FAST FACT

The number of eyelid surgeries performed in North America has increased by over 50% in the last ten years.

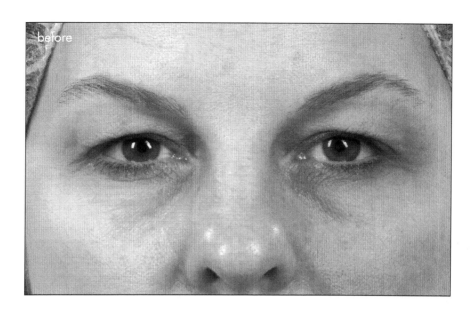

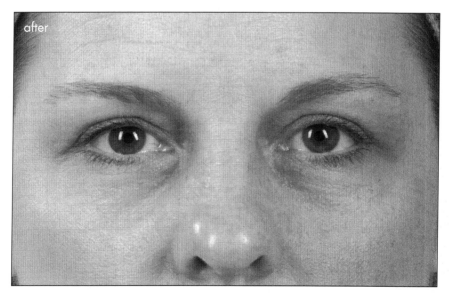

Upper blepharoplasty removed loose upper eyelid skin to allow for more exposure of the eyelid and a resulting less tired, more alert appearance.

these can be considered maintenance treatments. In other words, you can prolong the youthful look you achieve with your eyelid lift with occasional visits to your doctor to freshen up your eyes with one of these treatments.

★ FAST FACT

Because sagging eyelids can impair vision, your eyelid lift may be covered by your health insurance.

What am I going to look like when it's all done?

Your eyelid lift can create more sculpted eyelids that can take years off of your appearance. Your eyes can more easily express what you want them to express.

A skilled surgeon will take the time to discuss exactly the type of look you want to create and recommend looks that are appropriate for your facial structure.

Another great aspect of eyelid surgery is that scarring is often minimal because the incision is placed in the natural crease of your eyelid.

In the weeks after your procedure, the location of your incision can be slightly red and raised, but as the scar heals, it tends to fade.

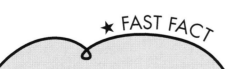

★ FAST FACT

If you've had laser vision surgery, you should wait six months before undergoing any eyelid procedures.

The results of your eyelid lift are usually long-lasting. Some patients ask for touch up surgery several years down the road, but many experience permanent results that last a lifetime. The permanence

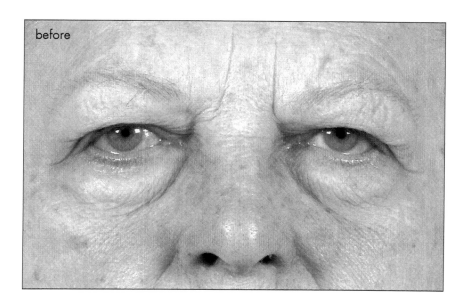

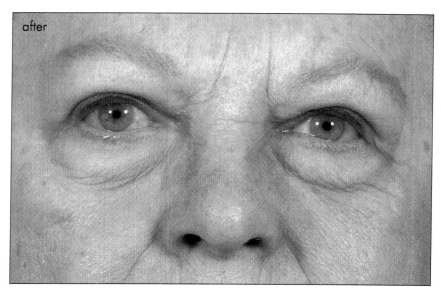

Upper eyelid lift with brow lift. both procedures help to improve
heaviness around the eyes.

of your eyelid lift will depend primarily on how prone your skin is to overstretching, but most patients are extremely satisfied with the longevity of their eyelid lifts.

Q & A WITH DR. KOTLUS.

Q **Will I experience changes in vision? How long will they last?**

A If an upper eyelid lift is done for functional reasons, when you may be covered by insurance, it's expected that there'll be an improvement in vision. Peripheral vision will become wider because we're moving the skin that's getting in the way of your peripheral view. For cosmetic upper eyelid procedures, the vision may change for a couple of reasons. Occasionally the eye will become drier after the procedure and you'll need some type of lubrication temporarily. Other changes in vision after the upper eyelid or lower eyelid procedure would be very rare, and they can be treated or addressed by your doctor.

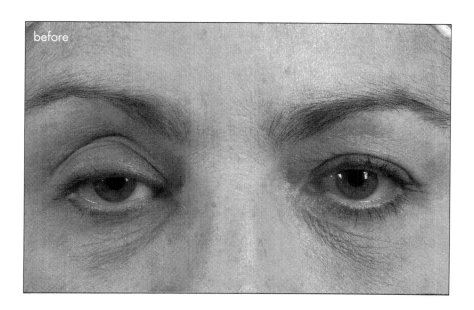

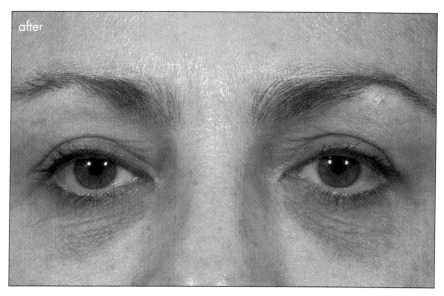

Repair of right upper eyelid ptosis (droopy eyelid) and filler placed under the tail of the brow to reinflate and lift the area.

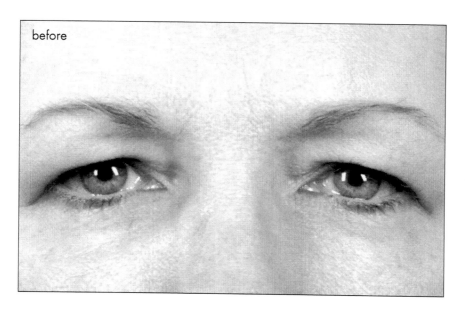

before

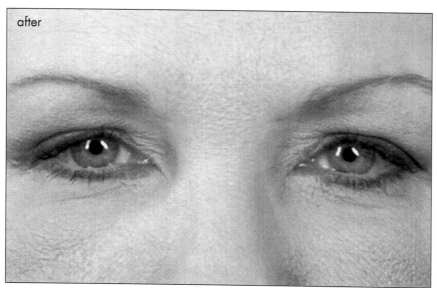

after

A brow lift in conjunction with an upper blepharoplasty creates a more
youthful look by elevating sagging eyebrows and removing extra
skin at the same time.

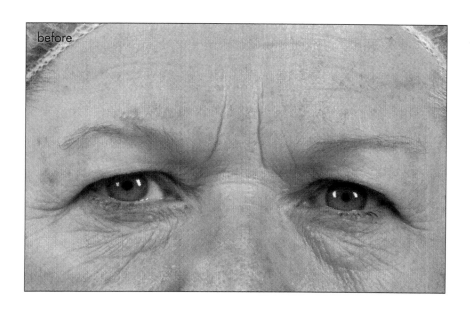

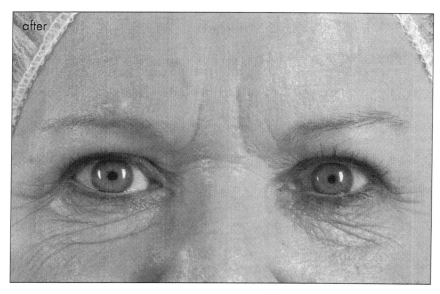

Both the brows and eyelid skin can contribute to tired-looking eyes.
Lifting both creates a more alert appearance.

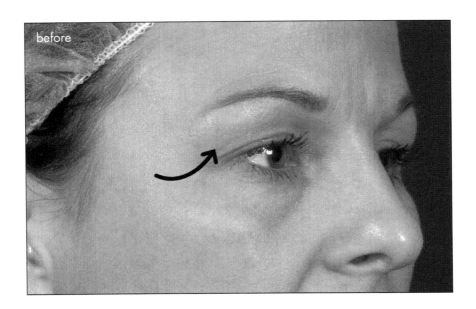

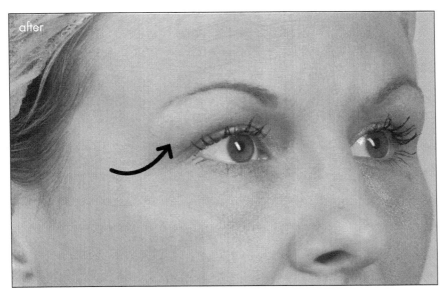

Fat transferred from the abdomen to the brow creates lift and a youthful contour without the need for a surgical brow lift.

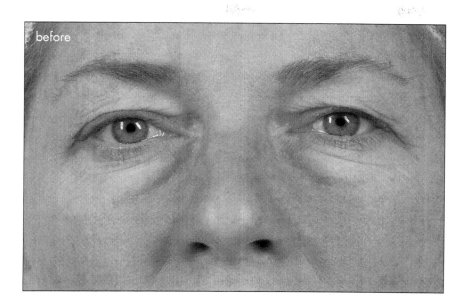

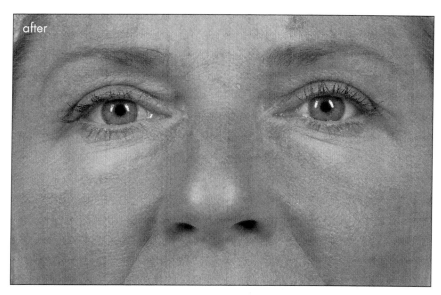

Upper blepharoplasty removes loose skin from the upper eyelids, creating a happier, younger appearance.

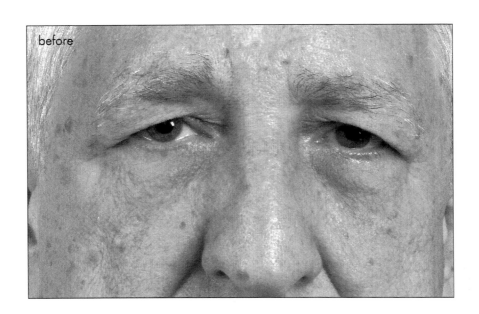

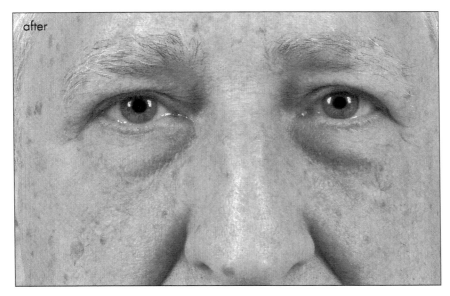

By removing droopy upper eyelid skin, this gentleman looks younger and has improved peripheral vision.

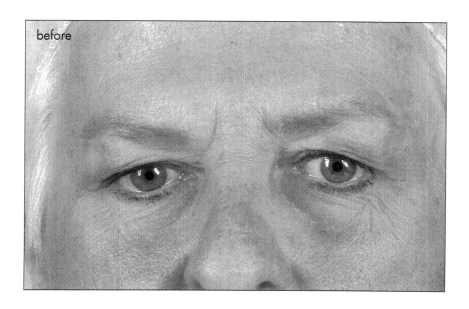

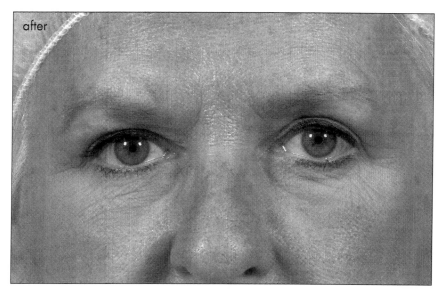

Removing extra skin with an upper eyelid lift allows for a place to put her makeup.

★ HOW ONE MAN GOT AN EYELID LIFT - AND A WHOLE NEW VIEW!

Gino works in construction and had so much puffiness and sagging around his eyes that it was impeding his vision and reducing his facial expressions. He had upper and lower bleph surgery and a cheek filler.

In the last three or four years, my upper eyelids had begun stretching to a point where it started to obstruct my view. Because of the puffiness above the lid, I couldn't open my eyes completely. I would have to actually physically raise my head up in order to have full view. It became obvious in my expressions and people noticed it, my friends and family especially noticed it. My family suggested that maybe we should do something about it.

I was a little concerned about what might happen with my face or eyelids; I wasn't sure what the ultimate outcome of this would be. And I work in construction, I work outside, so I was worried. Do I have to take some time off, will it be necessary to lose some time at work as a result of the operation? But I just lost a day; it immediately started healing. It wasn't a problem at all. Immediately after the surgery, the doctors said that everything went well. My face was covered up pretty good, so I couldn't see any results, but I was pleased. I knew that if they were pleased, then I was pleased.

Like I said, I went back to work the next day. You might feel self-conscious about how you look, kind of like you have a black eye. In my case, I didn't care. The doctors were a little

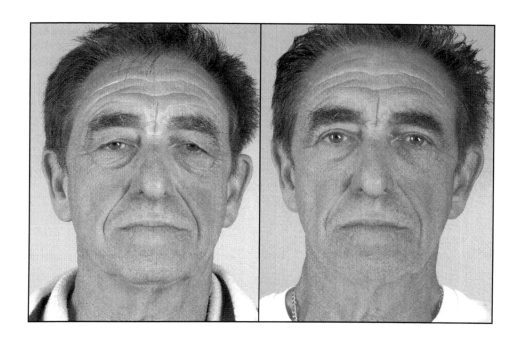

concerned that something might get in my eye, or that I might bump it or bruise it and that would create another problem. But I was very careful about that; I wore sunglasses and I backed off the physical work and I was fine.

Before the procedure, in order to look directly ahead, I would have to elevate my head. Because of the puffiness my eyelids looked half closed. Now after the surgery, everybody's really noticed the fact that my eyes really open up. Now people notice my facial expressions, no doubt about it. It's a hundred and ten percent improvement! I have just about full view without raising my head. I was told that because the lines in my face are so deep that it can take more procedures to get the full results. At this point I haven't done it, but I do plan to go back for another procedure. If I had known what great results I would have, I would have done it sooner. I would recommend them highly- I've already referred a friend of mine and she's made an appointment with them. Both the doctors did a terrific job!

✔ CHECKLIST

☐ Which is best for me – an upper eyelid lift, a lower eyelid lift, or both?

_____

_____

_____

_____

☐ What will my eyes/eyelids look like after the surgery?

_____

_____

_____

_____

☐ When can I start wearing contact lenses again?

_____

_____

_____

_____

☐ What type of anesthetic do you use? What risks are associated with it? Is it possible to also get a sedative if I feel nervous before my procedure?

_____

_____

_____

_____

☐ What kind of discomfort can I expect during and after my eyelid lift, and how can I minimize it?

_____

_____

_____

_____

☐ When do I come back for a follow-up and/or to have any stitches removed?

_____

_____

_____

_____

☐ How long will the results last? Will I ever need a touch-up procedure?

_____

_____

_____

_____

☐ Am I a candidate to have my insurance company cover my procedure?

_____

_____

_____

_____

QUICK QUESTIONS: *Eyelids*

Is there anesthesia?

Yes, usually just a local anesthetic. Occasionally mild sedation is also used.

Where would the procedure take place?

It is usually done in an office or an out-patient surgical center.

How long will the procedure take to complete?

The procedure itself can last from thirty minutes to two hours. The length of the whole stay is usually one to three hours.

What is the level of discomfort I should expect?

The discomfort is minimal.

Will there be bruising?

There is usually bruising, but the degree will vary a lot depending on the patient. It usually lasts one to two weeks.

Will there be any swelling?

Swelling also lasts about one to two weeks.

Will there be any numbness?

Numbness is usually not an issue.

What type of bandages will I wear and when do the bandages come off?

There are no bandages for this procedure.

Are there any stitches?

For the upper eyelids stitches are used. These usually come out in about a week. Lower eyelid surgery may or may not use stitches. If stitches are used, they will also come out in about a week.

When can I go back to work?

You can go back to work the next day if you don't mind people seeing the bruising, but most people go back to work in about a week.

When can I start exercising again?

You should wait two weeks before resuming any extra-strenuous activity.

When can I expect the final result?

Patients usually see their full results within three months.

★ NOTES

★ NOTES

Chapter 2 ★

Solutions For A
Sagging Neckline

★ CHAPTER HIGHLIGHTS:

★ Genetic factors, the loss of collagen in our skin as we age, and gravity are all factors that can lead to a sagging, loose neckline.

★ Cosmetic surgery is the best way to get rid of that "turkey waddle."

★ Cosmetic neck lift procedures today utilize minimally invasive techniques whenever possible.

★ Neck lift procedures offer a more youthful, fresh appearance in the lower third of the face.

★ Neck lifts are permanent in that you may always look five to ten years younger than you would have without the procedure, although your skin may continue to lose collagen and be affected by gravity.

Can cosmetic surgery help my droopy neck?

Eventually, most of us end up with reduced muscle tone and excess flab around our chin line. Known to many of us as a "turkey neck," a sagging neckline can be a disheartening sign that you're getting older.

Cosmetic surgery procedures including liposuction and neck/face lifts may be the only way to get rid of that unsightly, wobbly skin that's hanging around your jaw line.

The youthful look and tone of our skin is determined by the amount of collagen in our skin cells. As we age, we lose collagen, which often results in poor skin tone and looseness. Add to that any damage caused by smoking, sun exposure, and not-so-perfect diets, and you've got a veritable recipe for an unwanted turkey neck.

Because your aging skin has likely been subjected to most of the above, a sagging neckline is often all but inevitable. This is especially true if you have weak muscle tone or have lost a lot of weight. Sometimes your skin and muscles will stretch so much that they simply can't rebound on their own.

Even if you've exercised and eaten well your whole life, you may still develop a droopy neckline due to a genetic predisposition. Some individuals simply have an unfortunate genetic tendency to collect fat in their necks as they age. In these cases, no amount of dieting or exercise can help you tone up your chin.

Of course, there's also the matter of gravity. Throughout our lives, everything on us is being pulled downward. As our aging skin loses strength, gravity pulls and stretches it, resulting in a tendency for our necklines to droop downward.

Thankfully, your cosmetic surgeon has a variety of options to help you deal with your sagging neckline.

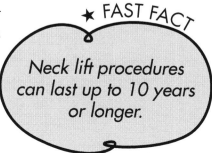

★ FAST FACT

Neck lift procedures can last up to 10 years or longer.

What are my options?

Various procedures are very effective in reducing your wobbly, loose neck skin. Your doctor can help you determine which one is right for you.

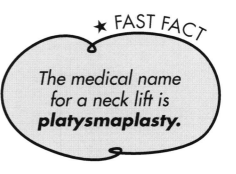

★ FAST FACT

The medical name for a neck lift is **platysmaplasty.**

Liposuction

Liposuction is a common technique designed to remove excess pockets of fat from beneath your skin. The procedure uses a cannula, which is a narrow, tube-like instrument inserted into tiny incisions made beneath the chin line. The cannula gently removes excess fat from your jaw line to reduce its saggy appearance.

A more modern treatment, called "laser liposuction," involves the use of a laser to enhance the procedure. The laser is carefully inserted under the skin through tiny incisions, then the surgeon gently passes the laser back and forth across your fat cells to break up any deposits, which makes them much easier to remove. Laser liposuction has earned a reputation for creating beautifully thinner, younger looking necks.

Both liposuction methods only take about an hour and create immediate and dramatic results in the look of your neck.

Platysmaplasty (neck muscle lift)

In many cases, sagging necklines are not actually caused by excess fat but rather excess skin or loose muscle. This can be especially frustrating to those of you who have worked hard to maintain a trim figure, yet still have the look of a flabby face and neck.

To correct these issues, a platysmaplasty – or neck muscle lift – can reshape the look of your neck with about two to three hours of surgery.

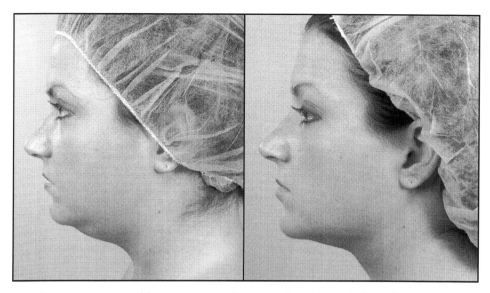

A small amount of fat removal underneath the chin with laser liposuction creates a nicer neckline with the appearance of having lost weight.

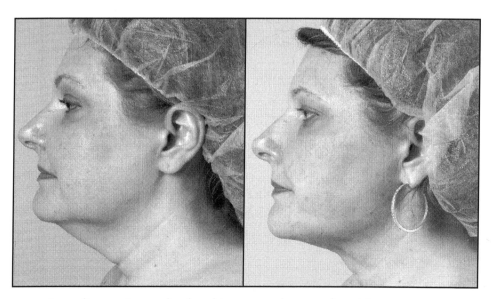

Laser liposuction under the chin removed excess fat while promoting modest skin tightening. She preferred this to the alternative of a lower facelift, as the mild muscle sag did not bother her.

This is a common option that will address any muscle bands or unsightly loose skin that have developed in your neck area over time.

This procedure involves a few small incisions under your chin and/or under and behind your ears, which allow your doctor to

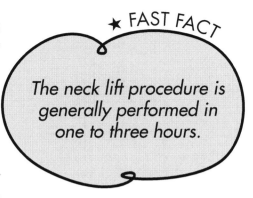

★ FAST FACT

The neck lift procedure is generally performed in one to three hours.

trim away or tighten the muscles on the underside of your jaw. Any loose ends can then be sutured into place near the front of your neck. At the same time, your doctor will gently pull any loose skin up toward your ears and suture it into place. The goal is a tighter, wobble-free neckline.

Rhytidectomy (lower facelift)

A rhytidectomy – or lower facelift – is a type of neck lift that also involves the lifting of your skin and tightening of your neck muscles. This procedure is often recommended if you have poor skin tone, overall muscle loss, or have lost localized muscle fiber tone in your lower face, jaw, and neck areas. The difference between a neck lift and a lower face lift is minor. In general, a lower facelift addresses the jaw line (jowls) and the neck, while a neck lift may simply treat the neck by itself.

The incisions for this procedure are carefully hidden around your ears, ear lobes, and in your hairline. Occasionally, your doctor may also require small incisions underneath your chin. Because your doctor will do his best to hide your incisions in hard-to-see places, visible scarring is usually minimal.

This procedure can take around three hours and can produce dramatic results in the overall look of your neckline by lifting droopy face and neck muscles as well as repositioning any saggy skin. Most candidates for a lower facelift enjoy a revitalized look that is both youthful and natural looking.

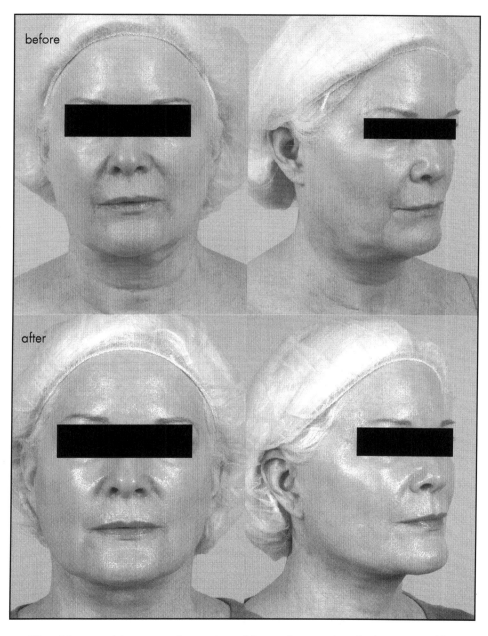

before

after

This 60 year-old patient always hated her turkey neck, which was just like her mother used to have. She had a lower facelift to improve the jawline and neck tightness. This makes the entire face appear younger.

Which procedure is right for me?

Before your procedure, you will have ample time to discuss with your doctor which procedure is best for your specific situation. In many cases, doctors suggest a combination of procedures to achieve optimal results.

Will my procedure hurt?

Most neck procedures are done under a local anesthetic known as "tumescent anesthesia." This anesthesia flows throughout your neck area. You will likely experience feelings of pressure, but actual discomfort should be minimal. Tumescent anesthesia also minimizes any bleeding during your procedure, which will help speed along your recovery afterward. General anesthesia is sometimes used in neck procedures, but it is often not required.

Anesthesia for the platysmaplasty – or neck muscle lift – is more involved. The tumescent anesthesia is usually circulated through your cheeks in addition to your neck area. In addition, you will likely have the option of having a sedative, which makes you drowsy enough to feel completely comfortable until the local anesthesia has made the treatment area completely numb.

If you do opt for sedation, you may also choose to be woken up during the actual procedure, which you won't feel thanks to the local anesthesia. If you'd like, you can communicate with your doctor throughout your procedure. If you're excessively anxious, on the other hand, you may be able to opt for sedation

★ FAST FACT

Neck lifts cause little discomfort with about a week's recovery time.

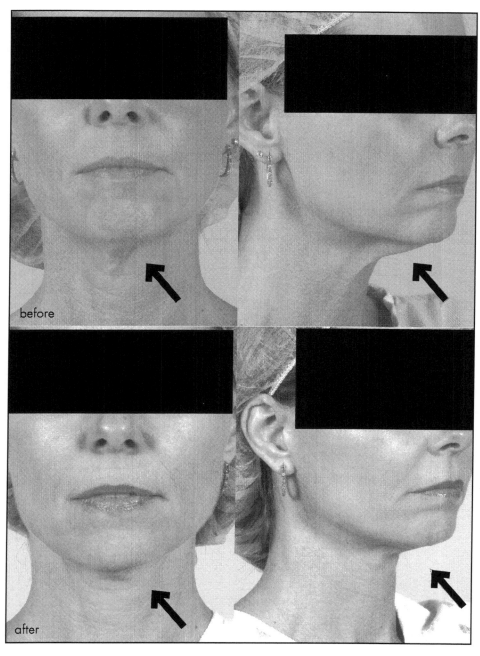

A neck lift improves a sagging muscle band seen under the chin.

throughout your procedure. Talk to your doctor about what you think will make you the most comfortable.

Overall, be aware that this procedure is painless for the vast majority of patients. Interestingly, many people report that laser skin resurfacing, which is actually less involved surgically than a neck procedure, involves more discomfort than any type of neck lift.

★ FAST FACT

Neck lifts can be combined with chin augmentation, laser skin resurfacing, eyelid, forehead, cheek, or brow lifts, and facial implants or fillers.

What about after my procedure?

Most people experience about a week of mild to moderate soreness after a neck procedure. You will likely be able to manage any discomfort you feel with an over-the-counter pain medication.

Swelling is also common after a neck procedure. You will probably find your neck the most swollen in the first day or two following your procedure, after which it will gradually subside. Your doctor will ask you to wear a neckband for your first week in order to minimize swelling, although you will be able to take it off occasionally if you'd like to go out without wearing it. After the first week, your doctor will likely ask you to continue to wear the neckband only at night for the next week or so.

Some patients also experience some mild to moderate bruising after their procedure. This will depend a lot on your individual physiological factors as well as things like diet.

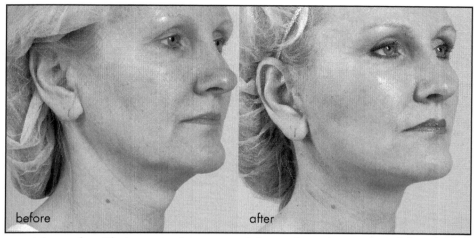

A lower facelift dramatically improved the jowls and central neck bands.
The incisions around the ear are nearly invisible.

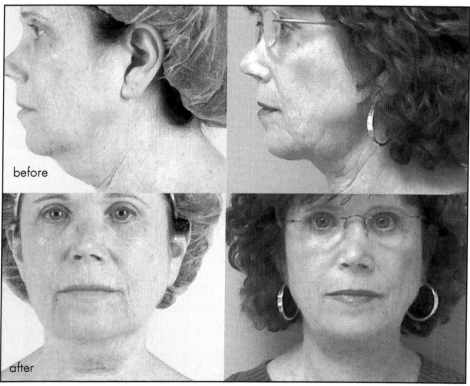

Before and after laser neck liposuction

It's normal for you to experience a degree of stiffness as well. You may feel as though someone is tugging on your skin – these sensations are perfectly normal and will likely subside. To reduce this type of discomfort, you can expect your doctor to ask that you minimize head movements for a couple of days following the surgery.

After a week, you should be able to resume normal activities, although it will usually take a couple of weeks for the swelling to settle down. When you return to work will depend on your individual comfort level. If you don't mind the outside chance of some of your more astute coworkers noticing you've had work done, you can go back to the office in about a week. If you're a little more self-conscious, you may want to wait for two to three weeks before returning to work.

If you've got a big event coming up where you want to look your best, such as a wedding, you may want to give yourself two to three months of healing time before the big day. Full healing can take several months, so you want to give yourself a large enough window of time to ensure you'll be looking your absolute best.

What am I going to look like when it's all done?

Because you will have had several small incisions, you can expect scars that will eventually fade.

Your new neckline often lasts about five to ten years. That means that, yes, you may have to return to your cosmetic surgeon if you want to maintain your youthful, wobble-free jaw line. This is because aging and gravity continue to do their work post-procedure. Your doctor can give you advice on what you can do to prolong

★ FAST FACT

A neck lift is performed in an outpatient setting.

the effects of your procedure, such as maintaining a good skincare regime, using sunscreen, and avoiding tobacco.

Some people like to think of it this way: if you had a twin that didn't have a neck lift while you did have one, you would always look five to ten years younger than your twin. In that sense, a neck lift lasts forever!

Q & A WITH DR. KOTLUS.

Q **What can I do to enhance and encourage the healing process after the procedure?**

A Having proper nutrition - a balanced diet low in fat and calories with plenty of fruits, vegetables, and grains - will help you to heal better. Your body's ability to regenerate skin and to heal wounds is enhanced by using multivitamins, maintaining good hydration, having a good amount of sleep. Your doctor could suggest antibiotics or topical creams to use after the procedure. Be sure to follow your doctor's instructions and recommendations closely.

★ HOW A MOM WENT FROM PHOTO-PHOBIC TO PHOTO-READY IN TIME FOR HER DAUGHTER'S WEDDING!

Grace had been so self-conscious about the loose, sagging skin under her neck that she refused to even have her picture taken. As her daughter's wedding approached, she finally decided it was time to do something about it- those were wedding photos she couldn't miss. It took Grace a couple tries to find a doctor she liked, but then she found Allure- and a new, more youthful neckline!

I had a lot of excess skin underneath my face and chin, and I just wasn't happy with the way I looked. Anytime someone would be taking pictures, I'd always shy away from the camera. And my kids would get upset- you know, Mom, they'd say, we really want a picture with you. And so I saw on TV the Lifestyle Lift advertised and I actually went in for consultation at a clinic about it. They told me at first they could do it, and then when I actually had a consultation with the doctor, they said, we can't do the Lifestyle Lift on you, but we could do this other procedure. It was like they said one thing when I talked to nurses and when I saw the doctor he said something quite different. He said it would be a big procedure, and they wanted to charge me quite a bit more money than they originally said, so I decided not to do it.

Then my daughter actually spoke to a friend whose mother had had a neck lift. She said she had gone to Allure and had a procedure done and she was very happy with it. So I thought why not give it a shot? I had a consultation at Allure,

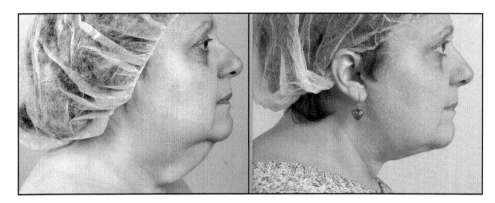

and I was very comfortable with Dr. Kotlus. And a lot of the girls who work there have had procedures done, and everybody's results look really good. I was very impressed with their honesty.

The thing that really pushed me to actually do it was my daughter's wedding. My daughter kept saying, 'I want you in the wedding pictures.' I had it done between the shower and wedding, so there wasn't a whole lot of time in between, and she was a little worried about me having surgery. But I knew this was something that I wanted to do for myself. My daughter got married a month after my procedure and people just thought I looked really good- nobody knew what I had done. I took a week off work. I didn't tell anybody that I had anything done but when I went back people were saying, 'Did you lose weight? Something looks different.' It was pretty dramatic- they just thought I looked really young.

I really didn't have any problems. You hear about facial surgery and about people having a lot of pain, but the only problem I had was trying to sleep upright. You have to sleep in a chair for a while. I did have a little bit of a scar but Dr. Kotlus took care of that with an injection. He was wonderful, he said 'I'm not happy with this,' even though the scar was pretty much covered with my hair and I thought it looked pretty good. He gave me a shot and it took care of the scarring. I was told by the nurses and I agree, he's a perfectionist- which is nice. You really know he's worried about what his finished product is. I'm very pleased and he was a very nice man. He is very thorough and he's just very caring- he's a wonderful doctor.

✔ CHECKLIST

☐ What type of neck lift technique or procedure do you recommend for my expectations and goals?

_____

_____

_____

_____

☐ What kind of anesthesia is used? Will I be awake during the procedure?

_____

_____

_____

_____

☐ What are the risks or complications of this procedure?

_____

_____

_____

_____

☐ Where will you be making incisions? Will I have scars?

_____

_____

_____

_____

☐ Will my neck line be smooth and toned after the procedure?

_____

_____

_____

_____

☐ How can I minimize discomfort?

_____

_____

_____

_____

☐ How long will the results of my procedure last?

_____

_____

_____

_____

_____

☐ What happens if I don't like the results?

_____

_____

_____

_____

_____

QUICK QUESTIONS: *Turkey Neck*

Is there anesthesia?

A local anesthetic is used and sometimes mild sedation as well.

Where would the procedure take place?

In an office or outpatient surgical center.

How long will the procedure take to complete?

Liposuction only is usually about an hour. If a muscle or neck lift is also done the procedure can be up to three hours.

What is the level of discomfort I should expect?

Discomfort is minimal. During the procedure patients will not feel any pain, although there may be some mild stiffness or soreness for about a week afterward.

Will there be bruising?

Some patients have no bruising, but others experience mild to moderate bruising.

Will there be any swelling?

There will be some swelling in the days following the procedure, but it should subside. Patients wear a neckband to help reduce it.

Will there be any numbness?

In some cases there can be numbness for a few weeks near the incision area, but everyone's experience will be a little different.

What type of bandages will I wear and when do the bandages come off?

Patients have a neckband that they will wear most of the time for the first week, and then just at night for another two weeks.

Are there any stitches?

For liposuction only no stitches are used. With the neck muscle lift and lower face lift stitches are used. They are removed about a week after the procedure.

When can I go back to work?

Most patients, however, go back to work about a week after laser liposuction and one to three weeks after a neck lift.

When can I start exercising again?

You can go back to full activity after two to three weeks. Avoid strenuous activity the first week.

When can I expect the final result?

You should be completely healed within three to six months.

★ NOTES

★ NOTES

_____
_____
_____
_____
_____
_____
_____
_____
_____
_____
_____
_____
_____
_____
_____
_____
_____
_____
_____
_____
_____
_____
_____
_____
_____
_____
_____
_____
_____
_____
_____
_____

Chapter 3 ★

Facial Treatment Essentials

★ CHAPTER HIGHLIGHTS:

★ Facial treatment procedures are a way to freshen up one's face and reduce the appearance of fine lines and wrinkles

★ Avoiding the sun and not smoking are two easy ways to preserve the health and the appearance of your skin.

★ Laser resurfacing procedures help those with fine to moderate lines, with a laser taking away the top layers of the skin.

★ BOTOX® (and Dysport®) injections are used for the elimination or softening of expression lines.

★ Dermal fillers help to fill in scars and lines on the face

★ Dermabrasion and microdermabrasion both work to 'sandpaper' off the outer layers of the skin to reveal younger and smoother skin.

★ Most facial treatments require little to no recovery time, although laser resurfacing and chemical peels can take up to fourteen days to heal.

★ Some facial treatment procedures need to be repeated at regular intervals for the best results.

What can a facial treatment do for me?

For many people, the march of time takes place on their faces first. If you find yourself wishing that Mother Nature wasn't quite so harsh to your face, you'll be happy to know there are a lot of simple facial treatments out there to help you take that step back in time, enough to fool even your harshest critic – yourself.

Although facial lines seem to come out of nowhere, there are actually two different causes for their appearance: environment and genetics.

Environmental factors – such as sun exposure, smoking, and tanning beds – damage your skin in a variety of ways (although they seem like a good idea at the time). However, even those of you who have avoided these skin-damaging habits may still fall victim to facial lines. Some families are simply genetically predisposed to have more lines than others, with generation after generation inheriting the same wrinkles as their parents and grandparents.

As age creeps up on us, this damage turns into lines and wrinkles that tend to deepen and lengthen over time, making them impossible to cover with makeup or so-called "skin smoothing" creams. These lines can make you look angry, tired, or sad all the time, which can negatively impact your self-confidence.

What to do?

Thankfully, there are a variety of options available to minimize or eliminate the appearance of facial lines. Smoother, more youthful skin is no longer a privilege only for the

★ FAST FACT

In 2007, approximately 42% of all non-surgical cosmetic procedures were BOTOX® injections.

young. With as few as one short treatment, your mirror could be showing you a fresher, smoother face that makes you look as young as you feel.

What are my options?

The most common signs of an aging face are:

- ★ Crow's feet around your eyes
- ★ Folds that run from your nose to your mouth (nasolabial folds)
- ★ Marionette lines from the corners of your mouth to your outer chin
- ★ Little lines around your mouth (periorial lines)

To combat these facial lines, you have a number of options at your disposal. Your doctor will help you choose the right treatments depending on the depth and locations of your lines.

For fine to moderate lines and wrinkles:

If you have fine to moderate lines, resurfacing laser procedures offer a quick solution. Two popular types, CO2 laser resurfacing and Erbium laser resurfacing, create small injuries to your skin that stimulate new collagen growth. The new collagen then tightens your skin, resulting in a face that can look years younger.

Some forms of laser resurfacing remove the outermost layer of your skin, allowing for a smoother, fresher face to reveal itself. The newest forms of laser resurfacing are fractional, which means they leave some of your outer skin layer in place. This option gives you excellent rejuvenation with less downtime.

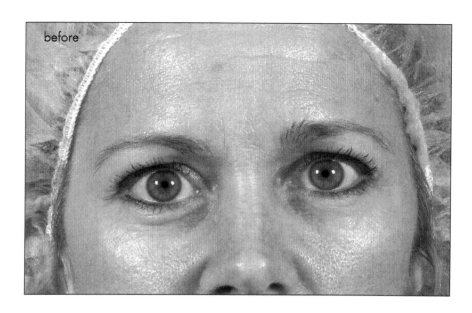

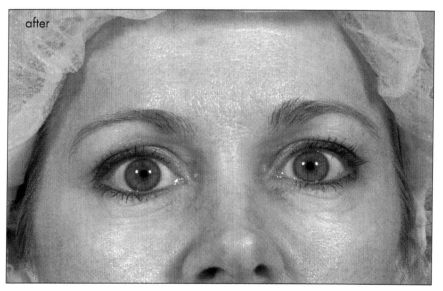

This patient received BOTOX® between the brows and at the outer corners of the eyes to smooth brow and forehead lines and create a less tired and more alert appearance.

For deeper wrinkles and expression lines:

Bothersome expression lines need a more targeted approach than your finer lines. For these, BOTOX® is one of the most effective and affordable treatments available; its popularity is well deserved.

BOTOX® injections help by relaxing your facial muscles, which smoothes the lines that are caused by the expressions you make. BOTOX® can be used on a regular basis, which means it's a great option for staying on top of any new wrinkles that turn up uninvited.

You do have options beyond BOTOX®, including a newer product called Dysport®. Similar to BOTOX®, Dysport® is currently available in the U.S. and many patients are seeing pleasing results. Your doctor can help you decide which product will work best for you- both of these products consist of botulinum toxin type A, so they work in the same way to reduce lines.

For deeper wrinkles and facial imperfections, dermal fillers are another effective option. These materials are injected into a targeted spot to plump up those lines and create that smooth skin surface you desire. As a general rule of thumb, BOTOX® is fantastic in the upper face (the forehead and around the eyes) while fillers tend to be most effective in the lower face (lines around mouth and nose).

To improve your skin's texture:

Chemical peels and dermabrasion can help you conquer an aging face by improving your skin's texture and giving it a smoother appearance. Ideally for those without deep wrinkles, these milder treatments help to freshen you up without any dramatic change.

Chemical peels work by applying chemicals to your skin for a period of time, which removes the outer layer and reveals younger and fresher skin underneath. A word of caution: peels can do damage when not administered by a qualified practitioner, so make sure you choose an accredited, experienced professional to perform your chemical peel. Alternatively, ask your doctor about laser resurfacing (see above), which provides the same

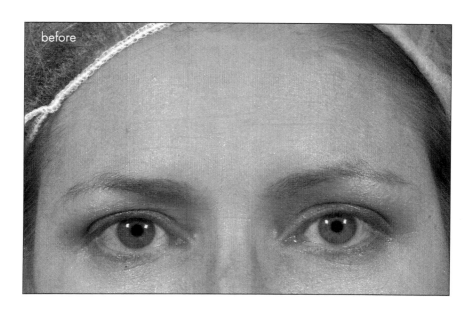

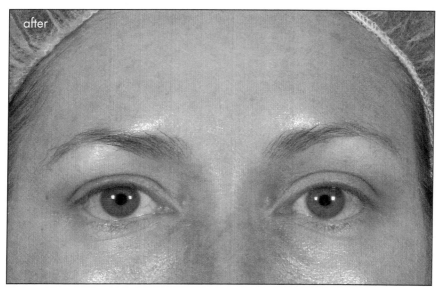

Before and 2 weeks after BOTOX® treatment around the eyes. Relaxing these muscles creates a nonsurgical brow lift.

effect and is considered to be safer.

Dermabrasion is essentially a sandpapering of your skin's outermost layers, which removes your most unsightly skin so that new skin can take its place. Because this treatment is designed to improve your skin's texture, it works well if you have facial scars you would like to minimize.

Microdermabrasion, dermabrasion's milder cousin, is a treatment that only removes dead skin cells. This can freshen you up in a snap, although because it is so mild, it's usually best as a maintenance treatment between more effective facial procedures.

Will my treatment(s) hurt?

Pain is a common concern, especially with facial procedures. Your face is filled with sensitive nerve endings, so you'll want to discuss with your doctor what pain, if any, to expect during treatment.

Most facial procedures use a local anesthetic, especially injection treatments (such as dermal fillers). Local anesthetic involves a small injection to freeze the treatment site so you won't likely feel much other than the initial anesthesia needle. The needle itself is generally very small; you'll probably only feel a slight pinch.

Topical anesthetics are occasionally used in these procedures, as well, so you may have an alternative to local anesthetic. If you're particularly squeamish about needles, talk to your doctor about topical anesthetics or other options.

With dermabrasion and chemical peels, you'll be exposing new skin, which means you can expect a degree of pain. Your personal level of pain tolerance will play a role here. Laser resurfacing, on the other hand, is relatively pain-free; again, talk to your doctor about what to expect and what will work best for your particular facial issues.

The good news is that even if there is a little pain (and usually it really is only a little), these are all relatively quick procedures. That means you won't have to bear any pain you experience for long and your doctor will do his utmost to keep you as comfortable as possible.

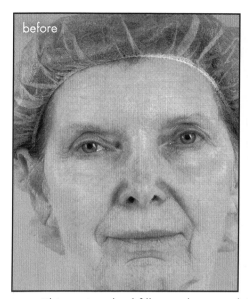 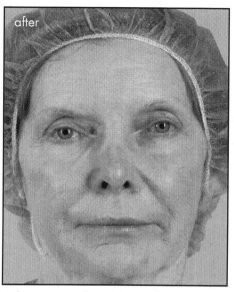

This patient had fillers to her nasolabial crease and marionette lines to soften her deep expression lines.

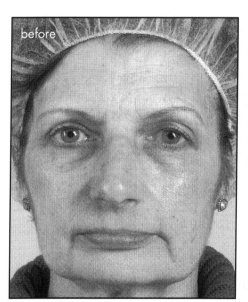 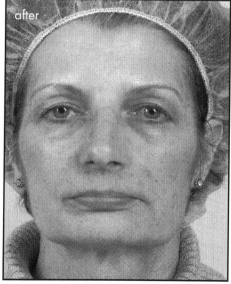

This patient had fillers to her marionette lines to reduce the shadows at the corners of her mouth.

What about after my facial treatment?

With some facial procedures, you can return to work the same day. BOTOX® injections, for example, take just five minutes; you can be back at the office after a lunch hour appointment.

More involved treatments – such as skin resurfacing, peels, and fat injections – may require seven to fourteen days of healing in order to be ready to be shown off to the world. These treatments are designed to selectively injure damaged skin, so you'll likely experience redness between the procedure and the end result. Your doctor will let you know exactly what to expect.

In order to minimize the recurrence of your wrinkles, it's best to avoid the two biggest skin-damagers: smoking and tanning. Smokers tend to have less skin elasticity and thus begin to show their age far earlier than non-smokers do. In addition, use at least a 40 SPF sunscreen whenever you are out in the sun, and reapply often. Wearing a large-brimmed hat will also help protect you from those damaging rays.

A little protective care for your skin will go a long way in prolonging your facial treatment. Avoid smoking and tanning and you'll enjoy your younger-looking face for as long as possible.

Using a good topical skin care regimen including a vitamin A product (retinols) and a vitamin C product can help prolong the benefits of skin treatments, and your doctor will make suggestions about products for you.

What am I going to look like when it's all done?

If you started off with moderate wrinkles, you will usually notice a significant change in the depth of these lines. If your lines were very deep, however, it might be impossible for any surgeon to completely erase them from your face.

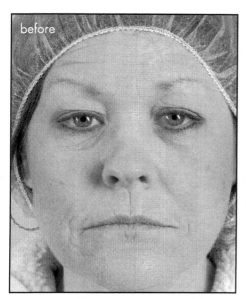 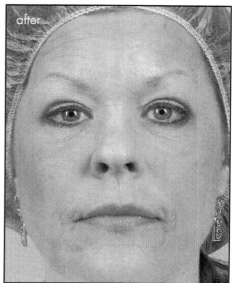

This patient received laser resurfacing to smooth the skin,
while fillers fill in creases.

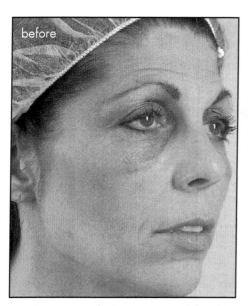 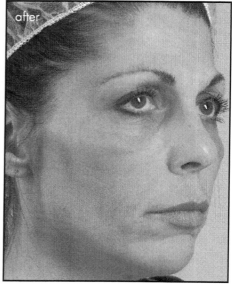

Laser resurfacing was used for this patient to tighten the skin and reduce
lines, while BOTOX® lifts the brow to a more relaxed position.

BOTOX® used on expression lines tends to produce the most dramatic results. Although the procedure takes only a few minutes, you will likely notice substantial improvement in a few days. Most patients report looking fresher, more awake, and far more youthful than they did before.

What's interesting about facial treatments is that while some have an immediate effect (like dermal fillers), others take a few days to really show their results (like BOTOX® and Dysport®). For example, when you remove layers of skin with lasers or peels, you need to wait a few days for the new skin to grow in.

How you have treated your skin in the past and how you care for it post-treatment will affect the success and longevity of your procedure. Keep in mind that no facial treatment is permanent, so if you want to keep your new youthful look, you'll likely need follow-up procedures at regular intervals. Your doctor should let you know how often you'll need repeat treatments.

Q & A WITH DR. KOTLUS.

Q **How can I maintain my facial treatment results after the treatment?**

A Whether or not the procedure is done on the face, I always suggest that they avoid sun exposure and use sunscreen diligently. Then maintain a good skin care regimen, which in many cases would include moisturizing agents, anti-oxidants, and topical vitamin A and vitamin C.

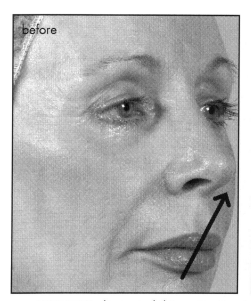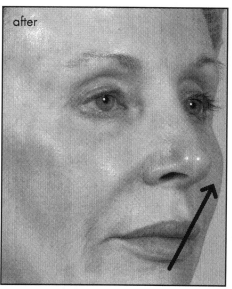

BOTOX® eliminated this patient's crows lines and helped her to appear
more alert. Filler to the cheeks created a smoother, younger shape.

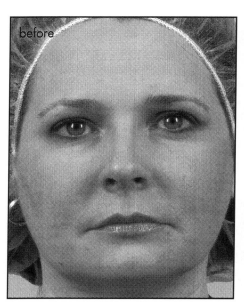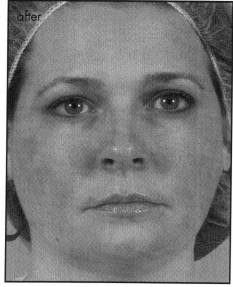

before and after BOTOX® around the eyes to create a more alert
but natural appearance

✔ CHECKLIST

☐ Am I a good candidate for a facial treatment?

_____
_____
_____
_____

☐ What are the differences between a laser peel and a chemical peel? How do I know which is right for me?

_____
_____
_____
_____

☐ Do I need to prepare my skin in any way before the procedure?

_____
_____
_____
_____
_____

☐ What are the risks of this facial treatment?

_____
_____
_____
_____

☐ Will I be able to be out in the sun after this treatment?

_____

_____

_____

_____

☐ Will I be able to wear makeup after the
procedure is done?

_____

_____

_____

_____

☐ How much pain can I expect during and after
the facial treatment?

_____

_____

_____

_____

☐ How many of these facial procedure have you
done in the past year?

_____

_____

_____

_____

QUICK QUESTIONS: *Facial Treatments*

Is there anesthesia?

Laser treatments usually start with a topical anesthetic cream. For injectable fillers, a numbing shot may be used.

Where would the procedure take place?

The procedure usually takes place in the physician's office.

How long will the procedure take to complete?

Many treatments, such as BOTOX® and fillers, can be done in just a few minutes. Laser or other treatments that cover a wider area of the face may take up to 45 minutes or an hour to complete.

What is the level of discomfort I should expect?

They procedures are all designed so that they can be tolerated, but there may be some discomfort.

Will there be bruising?

There is always a risk of bruising with injectables, but the risk is usually minimal and there are things that the patient can do to minimize these risks, such as avoiding certain medications. Your doctor will advise you about what you can do to minimize bruising.

Will there be any swelling?

Swelling can occur, most commonly with fillers and laser treatments.

What type of bandages will I wear and when do the bandages come off?

Usually, no bandages are used for these treatments.

Are there any stitches?

Stitches are generally not used with any of these facial treatments.

When can I go back to work?

Patients often go back to work the same day.

When can I start exercising again?

You can usually exercise within one to two days after treatment.

When can I expect the final result?

You should see good results within a week, although some of the laser treatments continue to improve in appearance over the period of a month.

★ NOTES

★ NOTES

Chapter 4 ★

All About
Your Breasts

CHAPTER HIGHLIGHTS:

★ Breast augmentation, reduction, or lift offer a solution to sagging, drooping breasts.

★ Three common procedures to deal with sagging breasts include breast implants (augmentation), a breast lift, called mastopexy, or breast reduction.

★ Your doctor has several options in deciding where to place the incision to minimize scarring.

★ You will be able to return to work within several days to a week after your surgery in most cases.

★ You should avoid vigorous physical activity and exercise for a few weeks after surgery to enhance the healing process.

★ Breast implants are typically made of saline or silicone.

★ Breast reduction may be covered by your health insurance.

What can cosmetic surgery do for my breast

Let's face it: women aren't always satisfied with the appearance of the breasts. Some women notice that, over time, their previously firmer breasts start to sag. Others are unhappy with the size of their breasts: sometimes they're too big, sometimes they're too small.

For many women, breasts play an important role in their identity and sense of self-confidence. It can be a little depressing to discover that breasts you once were proud of are now hanging much lower than you would prefer. It can be just as difficult when you are embarrassed by your cup size. If your breasts are too big, it can cause unwelcome looks and actual physical pain. If they're too small, you may not feel as womanly as you'd like.

As you have probably noticed, your breasts can change significantly in size and shape over the course of your life. Sometimes this happens after losing a significant amount of weight or having children. Sometimes it's a simple case of aging or unlucky genes.

Whatever your particular dissatisfaction with your breasts, there are steps you can take to rectify the issue. In most cases, a cosmetic surgeon can create the look you'd love to see in the mirror every morning. Cosmetic breast procedures are designed to lift, plump, or reduce the size of your breasts.

What are my options?

Modern cosmetic surgery affords you several options to enhance the look and feel of your breasts. The option that's best for you will depend on the type of change you want to make as well as the exact look you're after.

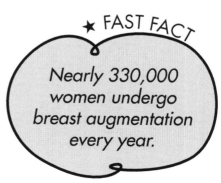

★ FAST FACT

Nearly 330,000 women undergo breast augmentation every year.

he look of your best ... with saline or ... gels are most commonly used in breast augmentation procedures.

Usually, either type of implant will consist of an outermost layer called the shell, mandril, or envelope, as well as the filler of your choice. There will also be a patch or valve that covers the area on the implant where the filler has been inserted.

In the U.S., the most common implants are saline pouches. This sterile salt water- or IV-type solution is placed inside a silicone rubber shell. The other type is the silicone implant, which has been gaining in popularity since it was reintroduced into the cosmetic surgery market. Silicone implants are filled with a soft, elastic gel that is described by some cosmetic surgeons as having a texture and consistency similar to that of a soft gummy bear.

Silicone gel is less likely to produce ripples or scallops around the edges of the implants. This bumpiness can sometimes be seen through your skin, especially if you have thin skin or a small amount of breast tissue to start with. Because silicone gel implants reduce the likelihood of visible ripples and have a more natural feel, they are considered more of a "deluxe model" over saline pouches.

Breast implants can have rounded surfaces or can actually be customized with various shapes and textures. Average sizes range from 120cc to 850cc (milliliters) in volume. Your body type and desired look will help you and your surgeon decide which type and size of implant is right for you.

During your actual procedure, your surgeon will make an incision in each breast to insert your implants. The actual location of your incisions will vary depending on where you're having your implants placed.

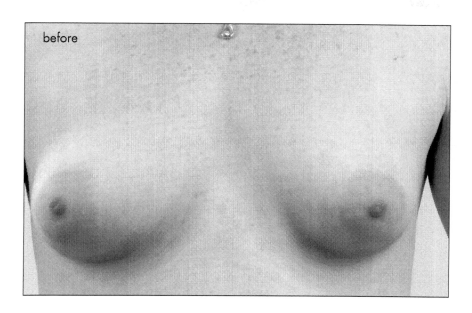

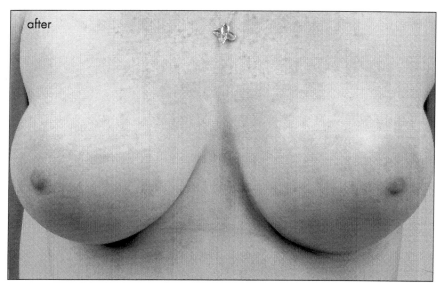

This patient's implants were placed through the armpit to create volume and restore symmetry. The photo in the lower half was taken one year after her surgery. The armpit incisions are nearly invisible.

Your options for implant placement are normally:

★ **Sub-muscular** – implants are placed under both your breast tissue and your pectoral (chest) muscles

★ **Sub-glandular** – implants are placed under your breast tissue but on top of your pectoral muscles

★ **Sub-fascial** – implants are placed under your breast tissue and inside of the pectoral muscle lining

★ **FAST FACT**

Breast reduction is also known as reduction mammaplasty.

The incisions for breast augmentation can be placed in one of four locations: under the breast, around the nipple, in the armpit, or around the belly button. These scars fade over time. The decision about which incision to use is based on your preference and your doctor's experience.

Breast lifts

Droopy breasts are often corrected using a procedure known as mastopexy, more commonly known as a breast lift. This procedure raises breasts into a more youthful position by using various techniques that improve the shape and contour of your natural breasts.

Your breast lift can be customized to your individual needs. The techniques used and types of incisions necessary will be determined by the amount of sagging, overall breast shape and size, the quality of your skin, and the size and location of the areola.

Incisions are commonly made in three areas:

★ **Around the areola** (doughnut-shaped)

★ **Around the areola and down from the areola to the breast crease** (lollipop-shaped)

★ **Around the areola and down, then horizontally along the breast crease** (anchor-shaped)

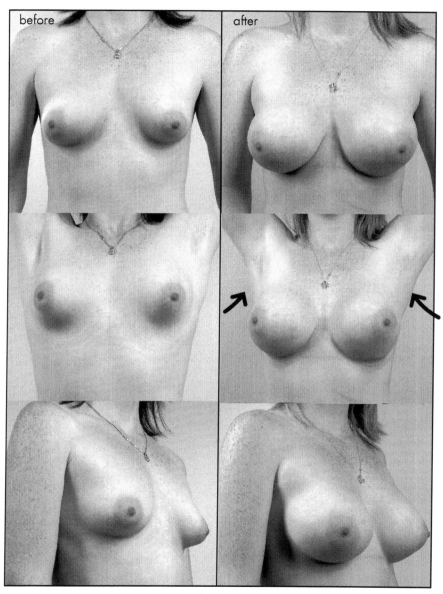

Breast augmentation with implants placed through the armpit. After three months, the incisions are almost invisible. Patient has nice increase in volume and appears more symmetrical.

Women with minimal breast sagging may benefit most from concentric – or "doughnut" – mastopexy. This procedure often requires fewer incisions. Circles that look like a doughnut are gently cut around the areola, through which excess skin and tissue are removed. A "doughnut lift" can have a tendency to stretch over time.

For women with lower breasts that require more lift, anchor- or lollipop-shaped mastopexy are two commonly preferred approaches. These procedures are often appropriate for women with larger breasts.

All of these techniques allow excess skin to be removed and the remaining skin to be pulled together, which creates a smoother, firmer appearance with less drooping or sagging. A breast lift may be combined with breast implants to create your desired breast shape.

Breast reduction

The most common procedure in a breast reduction is called the anchor-shaped reduction. Just like an anchor-shaped breast lift, an incision is first made around the areola. The incision then follows the natural curve of the breast to the crease. Through this incision, the surgeon removes excess tissue and fat to reduce the overall size of the breasts.

Because the nipples and areola are also in the area being reduced, they must be moved to a new position higher up on the surface of the breast.

A cosmetic surgeon may also choose to use liposuction to reduce the volume of the breast, often by thirty to fifty percent. This procedure can be done without scarring, but usually doesn't greatly enhance the overall breast position. Your doctor will talk to you about which options are best for your breasts.

Because excessively large breasts can be very heavy, painful, and actually cause damage to your body over time, breast reductions are sometimes covered by medical insurance. Talk to your doctor and insurance company to find out if you are a candidate for having your procedure covered.

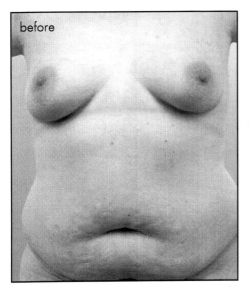 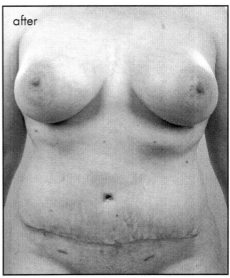

This patient had a combination breast augmentation with Combituck.
Often these procedures can be performed together so that the recovery
time is shared.

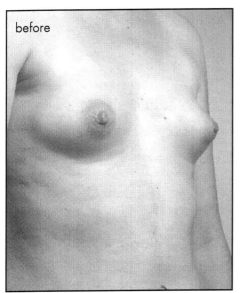 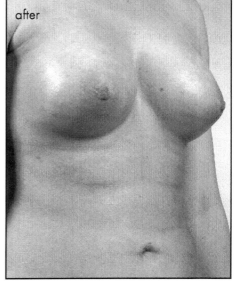

Saline breast implants placed through the belly button improved her
confidence without creating an unnatural look.

Will my breast procedure hurt?

With all breast procedures, anesthesia is offered in the form of intravenous sedation or general anesthesia, which means you shouldn't feel or remember a thing. Sedation is sometimes preferred over general anesthetic because it is milder and easier to "come out of" after your procedure is finished.

For most women, soreness or discomfort from any type of surgical procedure can range from mild to severe, depending on your individual pain tolerance. Whichever procedure you have, you can likely expect soreness in the breast area for several days. Most women can do light tasks as early as the day after surgery, but it may take one to three weeks to return to full activity.

Most women also experience some swelling of the breasts, which can also cause tenderness or discomfort. This is a normal reaction to the surgery and will usually disappear after a few days to weeks.

What about after my breast procedure?

Although it depends on the technique and type of procedure, your bust area will typically be wrapped in gauze and elastic bandages or a surgical bra following your breast surgery. In some cases, the bandages or bra may have to be worn for an extended time period.

★ FAST FACT

Roughly 150,000 women a year choose breast reduction procedures.

Keep in mind that you will need some recovery time in order for your swelling and soreness to completely disappear. After the period of healing is over, you will be able to see the full, finished result of your lift, reduction, or augmentation. This is when you will be able to fully appreciate the new size, position, and feel of your breasts. In very few cases, some patients have increased sensitivity in the breast or nipple area, though this is uncommon.

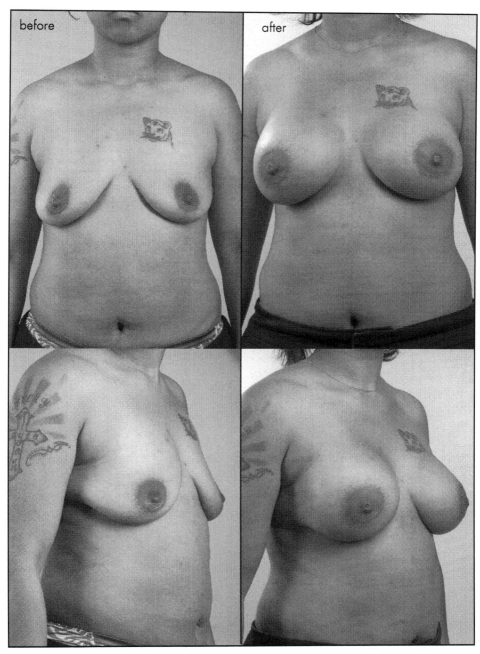

Breast implants placed through the armpit restored volume in this patient with multiple children. A lift was not performed, so there is no visible breast scarring.

If you've had a breast reduction, you will likely notice a greater freedom of movement thanks to the weight and volume that has been removed from your chest. Many women also report better posture and less back pain than they had with their uncomfortably large breasts. There are risks after breast surgery including scarring, implant deflation, loss of sensitivity, asymmetry, and hardening of the breast (capsular contracture). These issues can be discussed with your surgeon who can share information about the likelihood that these issues will arise and what can be done about them. In some cases, revision surgery is required.

> ★ FAST FACT
>
> From 2008 to 2009, breast reconstruction procedures increased by 39%.

What am I going to look like when it's all done?

Your end result will depend largely on your individual procedure. The goal is to achieve a natural look that balances the overall shape and proportions of your frame. Size isn't everything; your doctor will help you choose a look that is optimal for your chest structure.

Since your breast procedure involves incisions of some kind, you can expect some scarring. Your incisions will have been carefully closed with sutures, surgical tape, and/or skin adhesives, all of which will help minimize the appearance of any scars that develop.

The type of incision you have will dictate where your scars will develop. Some types of implant procedures can use incisions made in a crease in your armpit or even in your belly button.

If you've had implants, remember that it can take several months for the shape of your new breasts to look completely natural. This is because breast implants gradually settle into their pockets while the surrounding skin and muscle stretch and relax. Of course, you may also need some time to adjust to your new look.

Women undergoing any type of breast procedure are going to experience

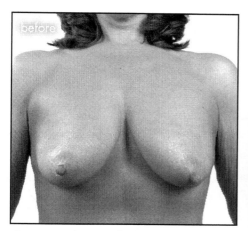 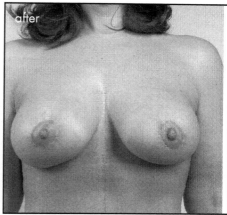

Breast implants with a concentric (or doughnut) breast lift improves the fullness and shape of the breast while raising the nipple to a more youthful position. The scars will continue fade with time. This photo was taken three months after the procedure.

enhanced self-esteem and confidence once their desired look is achieved. Your breasts are an important part of your overall appearance and the decision to get them just how you'd like is one that can make you look and feel like the youthful, vibrant woman you are.

Q & A WITH DR. KOTLUS.

Q **What will happen if I get pregnant after I have implants?**

A In the majority of cases, people can breast feed after breast augmentation. With pregnancy, the breast will tend to enlarge; you can develop stretchmarks as a result of this. The increased size of the breast can contribute to droop later down the road, so it's even more important to keep them supported during those times. But any woman can get pregnant after breast augmentation, usually without any negative consequences.

★ HOW ALLURE HELPED ONE WOMAN GET BACK HER BUSTLINE AFTER LOSING WEIGHT!

Julia, 46 years old, recently lost weight and found that as she did, her breasts lost volume as well. She had been so pleased with the results of the facial treatments she had done with Dr. Kotlus that she decided to get his help with improving her bustline as well.

I was unhappy with the way my breasts looked. I'm 46 now and I've lost probably 20lbs in the last year and when that happened I lost a lot of volume. I had gone to Dr. Kotlus before to get some filler done, and I did a laser skin rejuvenation with him. I thought he did such a good job with the filler. He's like an artist. I had seen brochures in his office about breast enhancement and at the time I thought maybe I was sagging a little bit, just from age, and he said, "No, you really aren't sagging. You've just lost volume"- from the weight loss.

My concern was that if I had an augmentation, it might alter my appearance. I thought I might end up cone-shaped or just something that didn't look like me. Dr. Kotlus reassured me that it would just be what I used to look like, and whatever size I wanted to go to. I know other women who have had implants but not with Dr. Kotlus. There's a gal at work, that's what you see when you see her coming. Boobs. I think she did that to balance out her look. But I am a tall and slender person, and given my body shape and everything I just wanted what I originally had.

I talked to him about the profile and the size and we did the 3-dimensional simulation. I wanted it to be a little

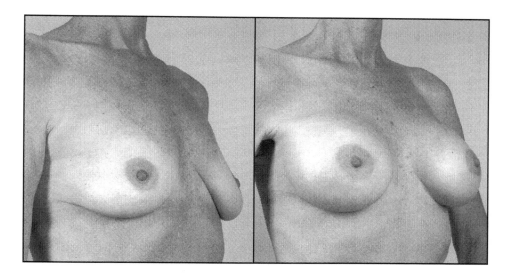

noticeable but I don't want to look like an adult film star either. And so he recommended 400 cc, and they're spectacular. They look so natural. I got the saline implants, and he never tried to talk me into the more expensive silicone. He went through my belly button so I wouldn't have any scars. I love them totally. When I've shown my girlfriends, and they've known other gals that have done it, they say they're the most natural-looking pair they have ever seen.

The recovery actually wasn't as bad as I thought it would be. Dr. Kotlus called me that evening, which I admire. I'd had nurses call for other procedures at times but when Dr. Kotlus called me, I thought that was impressive. I was moving just a little more slowly than usual, I think just adjusting to the weight of them. The procedure was just two days before Father's Day. I went to church and went out to dinner with my dad that day and they were a little sore, but I really just noticed it going from laying down to standing up. I didn't get any bruising, and in a few weeks I felt completely better.

I've told so many people about Dr. Kotlus. I didn't even look into other doctors. He made it seem like it's just a simple procedure anymore. He did such a great job. I just loved his manners; he was so calm and so professional and realistic. Seeing my results now, I would have it done sooner. I feel sexier than I ever have…and I'm 46!

★ EVEN HER OWN DOCTOR COULDN'T BELIEVE ONE WOMAN'S FANTASTIC RESULTS!

Zina had a breast augmentation and mesotherapy with Dr. Kotlus. Having seen results of breast augmentation that she didn't like, she was very concerned with getting the most natural look. Her results were so natural, even her own doctor couldn't believe they were implants!

I was always smaller than everyone else as a kid. When I grew up, it seemed like every part of me grew except my breasts. Also, I am a nudist. Even though after a while you're not self-conscious anymore about your size, you still see everyone else and you think, "Aw, I want that too."

There are some people down at the nudist campground that I belong to who have had breasts implants, but to be honest most of them don't look very good. So for three years, I didn't do it. Then, I did a lot of research. I even went to the hospitals in the area and asked the mammogram techs what they have seen. Well, from them I learned where not to go, but even they couldn't tell me about people who had had really good results. When I called different doctors, they couldn't tell me anything. They just said that they would have to see me.

At Allure, it was totally different. Everyone was so helpful. The people who answer the phones can actually help you. And if they can't, then they find someone who can. And when you're there, they act like you are the only person there. I don't know how they can schedule around that, but somehow they always have time to answer every question.

Originally, I was going to have a tummy tuck at the same time, but Dr. Kotlus told me, "you could do Mesotherapy

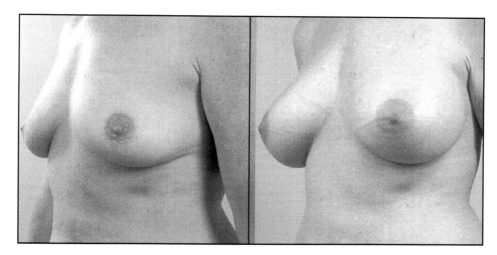

if you wanted to, but you just plain don't need a tummy tuck." I thought, wow, I was going to give you five thousand dollars but you've talked me out of it. They even had three girls come into the room and we were all comparing bellies.

I went to my regular doctor for my yearly checkup not too long afterwards and he was amazed. He inspected me and looked under my arms to try to find scars. It was funny. He's usually so shy and reserved, but he was literally playing with them. He had a ton of questions and he wrote down all the information about Allure. He said that women ask him all the time for advice about where to go and he had never been able to tell them. Now he can tell them about Allure.

Everyone has said I look great, but nobody could tell. It was the funniest thing. I went from an A to a C cup, but nobody could tell that's that what it was. They said I looked different and that I looked healthy. People thought that I had lost a lot of weight. But nobody could figure out exactly what the difference was until they were told. Nobody said, "Oh, you must have had work done."

I would tell anybody not to hesitate. Dr. Kotlus won't go any bigger than you should be. He'll follow the shape of your body, and he warns you what to expect ahead of time. With me, Dr. Kotlus said, "Yours are naturally far apart, and I can't move them closer together." He said that I didn't want to go too big because they would stick out under my armpits. He's so honest and straightforward with you!

✔ CHECKLIST

☐ What type of implants will be best for me and
my body shape and frame?

_____

_____

_____

_____

☐ What kind of discomfort should I expect?
Will it last long?

_____

_____

_____

_____

☐ How long will I have to stay out of work?

_____

_____

_____

_____

_____

☐ When can I resume my daily exercise routines?

_____

_____

_____

_____

_____

☐ Will I have scars?

_____

_____

_____

_____

☐ What are the risks to this surgery?

_____

_____

_____

_____

☐ Will my health insurance cover my breast augmentation/reduction/lift surgery?

_____

_____

_____

_____

_____

☐ How long will my breast implants last?

_____

_____

_____

_____

_____

QUICK QUESTIONS: *Breasts*

Is there anesthesia?

There is an intravenous sedation (IV) as well as local anesthesia.

Where would the procedure take place?

The procedure takes place in an outpatient surgery setting.

How long will the procedure take to complete?

The length of the procedure is approximately one to two hours. You are discharged typically about three hours after you come in.

What is the level of discomfort I should expect?

You should expect moderate discomfort. The first week will be the sorest time, but patients can walk around and go shopping. Initially you'll want to move your arms less and avoid heavy lifting. Soreness usually lasts around three weeks.

Will there be bruising?

Bruising varies, but it's usually not significant. About half the patients have mild to moderate bruising.

Will there be any swelling?

Typically there is swelling for the first or second week after the procedure, but it goes away quickly after that.

Will there be any numbness?

It's variable, but it's not unusual to be numb for the first couple of days. Sometimes there can be an area, like under the arm, that can be numb for a few weeks to a month, but it's usually a small area and it doesn't bother patients.

When do the bandages come off?

For the first night patients wear a special surgical bra and sometimes they have a type of strap holding things in place; those are usually removed after the first day or the first couple of days. They wear a surgical bra the first week and then switch to a different style of bra after that.

Are there any stitches?

It depends on the approach, but there are stitches. Usually they either under the arm or under the breast, and they typically are in for a week.

When can I go back to work?

After a few days most people can get back to work if you're doing "light" work. More active work usually requires waiting a week or two.

When can I start exercising again?

You can go back to full activity by usually within two to three weeks.

When can I expect the final result?

You'll see immediate results, but expect the final results in three to six months.

★ NOTES

★ NOTES

Chapter 5 ★

Dealing With Unwanted Fat

CHAPTER HIGHLIGHTS:

★ Mesotherapy, or Lipo-Dissolve, is a minimally invasive procedure effective in reducing small areas of fat.

★ Laser liposuction, also minimally invasive, is a procedure that ruptures and removes fat from localized areas of the body, most commonly the lower abdomen, thighs, and upper arms.

★ Tumescent liposuction is a treatment that minimizes bleeding and discomfort.

★ Excess skin removal tightens and improves appearance of areas where loose or stretched skin causes unwanted "pooches" or "bulges."

★ Fat reduction procedures offer positive and long-term effects when balanced with adequate exercise and diet.

Can cosmetic surgery help with my stubborn fat?

Excess fat is something almost all of us deal with at some point in our lives. Whether you're twenty, seventy, or somewhere in between, chances are you'll have unwanted fat deposits that just don't seem to go away.

This can be especially frustrating when you've made concerted efforts to eat well and exercise regularly. The unfortunate truth is that, no matter how disciplined you are, sometimes fat seems impossible to get rid of. Certain genetic and physiological makeups are simply more vulnerable to storing fat in the most unflattering of places.

The results of a busy lifestyle, compounded by your genetics and the natural process of aging, can result in a figure that frustrates you every time you look in the mirror. This can affect everything from your self-esteem to your personal relationships to your career prospects, but the good news is that you don't have to be stuck with that fat forever.

A variety of techniques and procedures are available today that produce excellent outcomes when it comes to fat reduction.

Of course, the best results will be achieved with a combination of cosmetic procedures and changes in diet and workout regimes. You should be aware that the purpose of cosmetic surgery is to help sculpt your body and is not a substitute for proper weight control. If you just have a bit of extra padding that you want to get rid of, your cosmetic surgeon can give you a head start.

The most commonly affected areas are around your hips, your thighs, and your lower belly. If you have fat in these areas, you may be a

★ FAST FACT

Nearly 500,000 individuals undergo liposuction procedures every year.

perfect candidate for a body sculpting procedure that can help you create the silhouette you envision for yourself.

While every doctor will recommend healthy changes to help you maintain your new, sleeker silhouette, you will probably notice an immediate boost in confidence that comes post-procedure. Often this new self-assurance is exactly what you need to encourage a new, healthier lifestyle.

> ★ FAST FACT
>
> Liposuction is listed as one of the top five popular fat reduction procedures in the U.S.

What are my options?

In most cases, methods used to achieve a nicer shape start with noninvasive procedures. If your cosmetic surgeon feels these treatments will be insufficient, he may recommend a minimally invasive procedure or something slightly more dramatic, if necessary.

Mesotherapy

Mesotherapy – also known as lipo-dissolve or injection lipolysis – is often effective in eradicating those smaller but troublesome areas of fat. Considered a non-surgical option for fat reduction, it is effective in cases where unsightly fat pockets appear and detract from your shape, even if you're thin.

Mesotherapy involves the injection of vitamins, pharmaceuticals, or natural extract agents under the skin. These treatments are designed

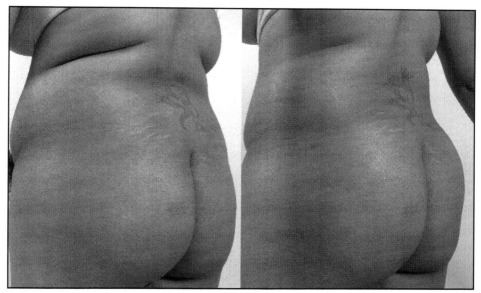

Patient had fat suctioned from flanks and hips and placed in the upper buttock, creating more roundness and projection. This is sometimes called a Brazilian butt lift. The photo on the right was taken nine months after the procedure.

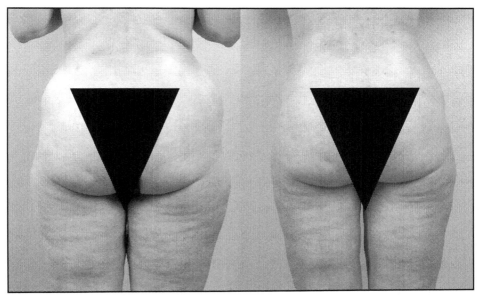

This patient had liposuction over several sessions because of the volume of fat removed. The patient lost weight at the same time, giving her an even better result with a much slimmer figure.

to dissolve fatty deposits and get rid of cellulite. The injections used include substances called phosphatidylcholine and deoxycholate, both of which have been proven to work well on small areas of fat. These substances act as detergents that damage fat cells so your body can eliminate them naturally.

This procedure is normally repeated multiple times, with each repetition improving your overall results. Mesotherapy works a little at a time, so you won't see an immediately dramatic change.

VelaShape™

Another procedure that is effective in improving the appearance of dimply cellulite is a process called VelaShape™, which uses radio frequency waves and infrared light. It offers between thirty and fifty percent improvement in the appearance of cellulite after about six treatments, each performed about a week apart.

Other similar radiofrequency devices are available that accomplish improvements in the appearance of cellulite. These non-surgical treatments give non-surgical results, which means they are less dramatic than a more invasive procedure but still create a noticeable change.

An Introduction to Liposuction

Liposuction is designed for fat removal and body sculpting, but not necessarily for cellulite improvement. The reason for this is that most women have a genetic predisposition for getting cellulite, which is determined by the way in which fat is configured under the skin. Strands of connective tissue between small fat pockets create the appearance of dimples, which may not be improved with any amount of liposuction.

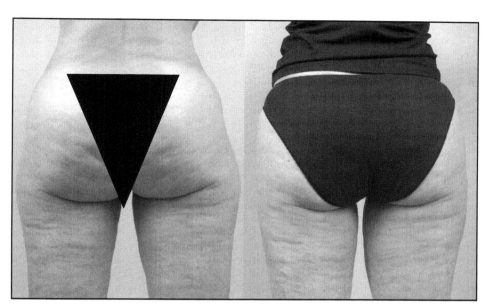

This patient had laser liposuction performed on the outer thighs to reduce saddlebags.

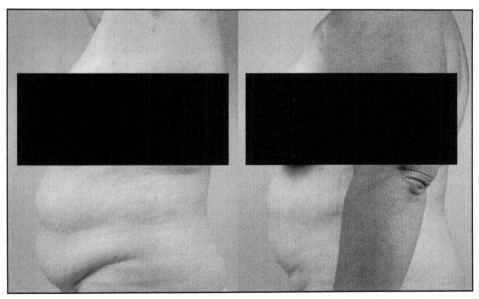

Liposuction can be used to remove the "pinchable" fat of the belly. The visceral fat, fat underneath the belly, must be removed with diet and exercise.

Tumescent liposuction

Tumescent liposuction got its name because of the type of anesthesia – called tumescent anesthesia – used during the procedure. Tumescent anesthesia is a fluid that is introduced into your target area, which increases the space between your muscle and fat tissues and simultaneously numbs the area. This additional space gives your cosmetic surgeon a greater range of motion to remove fat cells with small tubes called cannulas.

Tumescent fluid contains small amounts of lidocaine, similar to anesthetic agents used by dentists, as well as epinephrine, a medication that shrinks blood vessels to minimize bleeding and discomfort.

Tumescent liposuction also enables patients to choose between staying awake or being mildly sedated during the procedure. Although the procedure is painless for most people, some people feel more comfortable if they're under a mild sedation. This procedure takes between one and three hours, depending on your target area and the amount of fat to be removed.

Laser liposuction

Laser liposuction is a minimally invasive procedure that alters fat tissues by encouraging the rupture of fat cells, which are then easily suctioned out through a small tube called a cannula. Laser fibers are gently inserted into your target area and the energy emitted from these fibers causes your fat cells to rupture and drain.

This approach reduces bruising and promotes skin tightening as well as faster recovery time with minimal side effects. Laser liposuction is essentially a more modern form of tumescent liposuction, adding the

★ FAST FACT

*Americans spend about $13 **billion** dollars every year on cosmetic surgical procedures.*

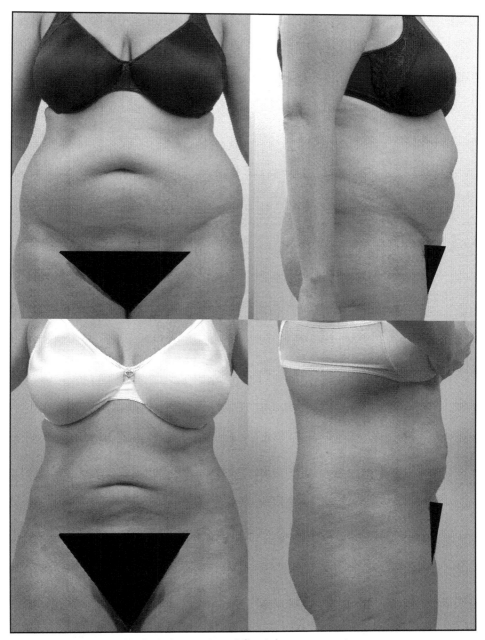

This patient had abdominal and flank liposuction. Liposuction can create a more proportionate figure, but additional weight loss will create a more slender frame.

laser to improve the procedure. Many surgeons achieve excellent results without the use of a laser, but the laser can make the job easier for your doctor and minimize any side effects for you.

Excess skin removal

Some individuals, such as those who have lost a great deal of weight or have been pregnant, are left with loose skin with poor tone, most commonly found in the lower belly area. In these cases, it is not excess fat that is the problem but rather excess skin and sometimes overstretched muscles. This excess tissue can create a silhouette that is just as stubborn and unflattering as those with unwanted fat deposits.

If you have an issue with loose skin or muscles, you may require a procedure that removes these excesses. Procedures like tummy tucks and brachioplasties (arm lifts) can firm up that skin and create a pleasing bodyline.

Excess skin removal procedures do normally produce some scars, but your doctor can often choose inconspicuous incision locations that will normally be hidden by your clothes. These scars will also fade over time. Talk to your doctor about your options for incision placement.

Will my procedure hurt?

Pain sensation will vary according to your personal level of tolerance, but in most cases you can expect to feel little to no discomfort during your procedure. Of course, you will also have some type of anesthesia and your doctor will make you as comfortable as possible during and after your procedure.

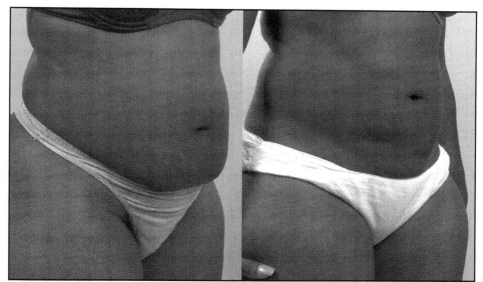

Tumescent liposuction created a nicer shape to her belly and sides, and lifted her hanging skin without a tummy tuck. The stretch marks remain, but her shape is much better and she was thrilled with the result.

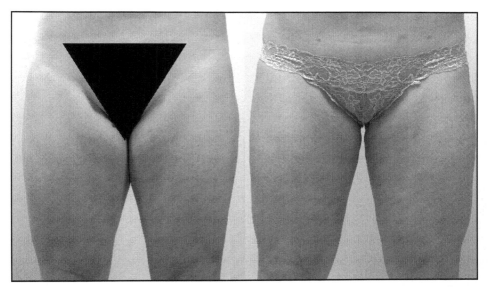

One week after laser liposuction to the lower abdomen and inner thighs. There is minimal swelling or bruising, and her inner legs no longer touch. The small openings through which the abdomen liposuction was performed are barely visible at one week, and will fade with time.

In addition to your personal threshold for discomfort, the type of fat reduction procedure you need as well as the surgical methods of your doctor will play a role in determining how much pain you feel. In surveys of post-procedure patients, however, nearly all agree that pain levels are tolerable and well worth the positive results they have achieved thanks to their procedure.

What about after my procedure?

Following liposuction, you will experience the most discomfort and soreness within the first two to three days. It's normal to be moving a little more slowly during this time. Some patients report that they feel like they've done a really tough abdominal workout in the case of abdominal liposuction, for example. Your doctor can recommend pain medication to help you minimize any discomfort you may feel.

Although heavy lifting and exercise should be avoided during the first week after your procedure, your doctor will likely recommend that you get on your feet and walk around as much as possible. After your first week of recovery, you will feel only minimal soreness that should no longer interfere with your daily activities.

After two or three weeks, you can likely expect to resume full activity, including exercise. From the day after your procedure until these two or three weeks are up, your doctor will have you wear a compression garment (clothing made of a form-fitting, stretchable material that squeezes the treated area) that will help minimize any swelling. He may also recommend massage therapy to help alleviate swollen areas as quickly as possible.

It may take between three and six months for your body to completely heal from your procedure, but this healing is primarily internal and shouldn't affect your ability to resume your everyday activities.

What am I going to look like when it's all done?

Most patients are overjoyed by their thinner, more flattering body shape. You may drop a dress or pant size or two and, of course, enjoy a boost in your self-confidence.

Of course, you should have realistic expectations before undertaking a fat reduction procedure. These techniques produce more or less permanent results, but remember that cosmetic surgery is not a substitute for proper weight loss techniques if you are significantly overweight. These surgeries are to deal with stubborn fat deposits that seem to persist despite diet and exercise. Under no circumstances should these procedures be treated as a substitute for a healthy diet and regular workouts.

If you have a lot of unwanted fat, it may be necessary to perform multiple surgeries (staging the removal of fatty areas over several treatment sessions). For safety reasons, it is not possible for your doctor to remove large excesses of fat all at once. Again, be clear about your expectations and be patient; your positive long-term results will be well worth the wait.

Once your desired silhouette is achieved, keep in mind that you will need to make an effort to maintain the changes your doctor has made, including any appropriate modifications to your food and exercise habits. Your doctor can advise you on what types of foods and exercise will be necessary for you to maintain your flattering new figure.

Treat your procedure as a long-term investment in your goal of a healthy, attractive body, and modify your lifestyle accordingly.

Complications are rare after liposuction. In rare cases, there can be extra fat left over or too much fat removed in a certain area. This can often be corrected with a touch-up when necessary.

Q & A WITH DR. KOTLUS.

Q **Will I have loose, sagging skin after my fat reduction procedure?**

A The most important part of any cosmetic procedure is selecting the right procedure for the right patient. So if someone has the tendency towards loose skin, where there's a lot of stretchmarks on the belly for example, then they might be a better candidate for a tummy tuck than they would for just liposuction alone. Loose skin that is pre-existing should be addressed with the original procedure.

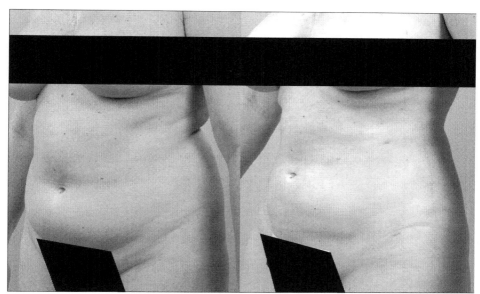

Liposuction contoured the belly pouch and 'love handles' that didn't seem to respond with diet and exercise.

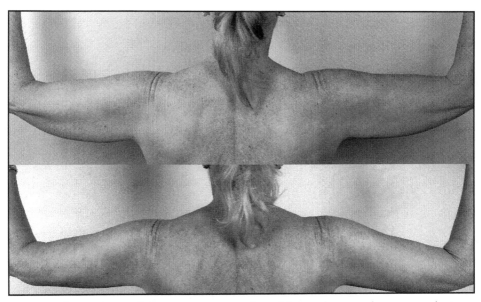

Laser liposuction of the upper arms reduced fat and created some modest skin tightening.

✔ CHECKLIST

☐ How much experience do you have performing Lipo-
dissolve/liposuction/laser liposuction?

_____

_____

_____

_____

☐ What type of fat reduction procedure suits my needs
and goals?

_____

_____

_____

_____

☐ What are the risks and complications of this procedure?

_____

_____

_____

_____

☐ What if the results are not as I anticipated?

_____

_____

_____

_____

☐ How large are the incision sites?

_____

_____

_____

_____

☐ What can I do to reduce any scarring?

_____

_____

_____

_____

☐ When I resume exercising?

_____

_____

_____

_____

☐ How long before I can return to work?

_____

_____

_____

_____

QUICK QUESTIONS: Unwanted Fat

Is there anesthesia?

Yes, typically IV sedation is used for liposuction.

Where would the procedure take place?

The procedure usually takes place at an out-patient surgical center.

How long will the procedure take to complete?

It will take one to three hours to complete the procedure, depending on the area of the body.

What is the level of discomfort I should expect?

There is moderate soreness in the week after the procedure. Patients are usually able to move around and do normal activities, they just move a little slower.

Will there be bruising?

It is not common, but occasionally there is bruising that fades in a week or two.

Will there be any swelling?

Yes, usually there is moderate swelling. Sometimes it can take a couple months to completely go down.

Will there be any numbness?

Some patients experience numbness, which can last for several weeks.

When do the bandages come off?

Patients wear a special compression garment for a few weeks after the procedure. This helps reduce swelling and provide support.

Are there any stitches?

Usually there are no stitches.

When can I go back to work?

Patients usually go back to work in about a week.

When can I start exercising again?

Light exercise like walking is okay to do the first week, and after two or three weeks patients are back to their normal routine.

When can I expect the final result?

You will see your full results in three to six months.

★ NOTES

★ NOTES

Chapter 6 ★

Wake Up Those Tired Eyes

★ CHAPTER HIGHLIGHTS:

★ Dark circles under the eyes and sunken hollows under the eyes can often be rejuvenated with minimally invasive procedures.

★ Injectable dermal fillers and/or facial fat transfer may provide that more youthful appearance you've been looking for.

★ Fat transfers are biocompatible, eliminating rejection concerns.

★ Injectable dermal fillers may include collagen, which gives skin strength and elasticity.

★ Injectable dermal filler procedures take an average of fifteen minutes.

★ Typically, dermal fillers and wrinkle smoothing injections are not painful and often require only local or topical anesthetic.

★ Fat transfers tend to be permanent, while wrinkle smoothing injections and dermal fillers may need to be repeated to maintain results.

★ Results of dermal filler injections can often be noticed immediately.

Can I do something about my tired-looking eyes?

Do you look tired all that time, regardless of the amount of rest you get every night? Many of us look in the mirror and are dismayed to see dark circles or sunken hollows under our eyes. The result is often a deflated vision of yourself, especially when you have no idea what happened.

A multitude of factors can contribute to a tired looking appearance. Consider the round, chubby face of a baby. Round, full faces equal youthful faces. As you age, naturally occurring pockets of fat in your face will shrink and lose volume, causing your cheeks to deflate and your eyes to appear sunken. These hollow spaces under the eyes can create noticeable shadows that look like dark circles.

In addition, aging eyelid skin tends to grow thinner and, in some cases, dark veins and muscle tissue just beneath the surface of the skin can become more apparent. Pockets of fat underneath the eyes, more commonly known as "bags," can also enhance the appearance of dark circles, make the lower eyelids look puffy and, unfortunately, make you look old and tired.

You are also constantly exposed to wind, sun, and other environmental factors like smoke, which take a toll on your skin. Even just using your facial muscles to make expressions can gradually deepen the creases on your face over time. These factors accumulate as you age and can negatively influence your overall appearance.

★ FAST FACT

Dermal filler injection results typically last about three to eighteen months.

What can you do to say goodbye to your tired eyes?

A simple cosmetic procedure may very well be the best solution for the circles, hollows or bags under your eyes. A fuller face gives a more youthful and toned appearance and, while none of us necessarily wants excess pockets of fat on our bodies, our faces are a little different. Procedures that enhance the fullness and volume of your face can give you a more youthful, fresh, and invigorated appearance.

What are my options?

The most common – and most effective – treatments to deal with tired looking eyes involve injections into the target area. These injections are often dermal fillers or transferred fat. Many people are also good candidates for BOTOX®.

These injections can plump up tired looking eyes and soften wrinkles or creases that are negatively contributing to the appearance of your eyes. Occasionally laser procedures are also recommended to enhance the overall look. Your doctor will discuss your options and help you come up with a treatment plan that works best for you.

Fat injections or transfers

Fat transfer procedures are becoming more popular every year. The major benefit of utilizing fat transfers is that they are biocompatible. This

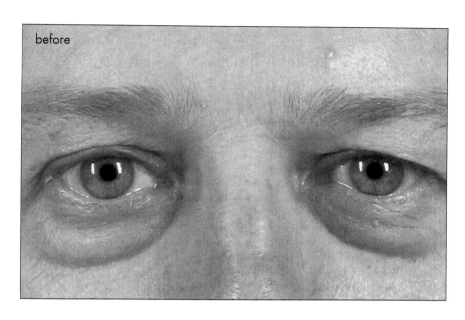

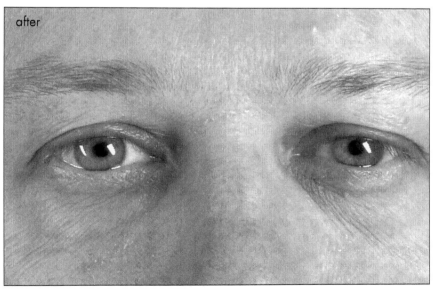

The bags of fat under this patient's eyes were creating a shadow which were making him look tired. By removing the fat, this patient has gained a more alert appearance.

means that the fat used to plump up the treatment area comes from your own body, so there are no issues with rejection, which can often be a concern in surgeries that involve tissue transfer from one person to another.

This type of procedure is often permanent because fat cells taken from one area of the body and relocated to another can stay there forever. An even greater benefit is that stem cells found in the transplanted fat cells tend to improve the overall health of the skin in that area, which can go a long way in restoring a youthful appearance.

The procedure itself is relatively straightforward. The fat is usually gently aspirated from a higher fat area (such as the belly or hips) on your body using a small tube. Next, the removed fat is injected into your under-eye area to restore lost volume and reduce the appearance of tired eyes. Sometimes the procedure must be repeated to achieve the desired result. In certain cases, the transformed fat is absorbed by the body, requiring another procedure.

Injectables: dermal fillers and wrinkle smoothers

Injectable dermal fillers are another popular alternative for facial enhancement, especially around the eyes. Some dermal fillers are not as permanent as fat transfers, which means you may need repeat treatments at regular intervals, usually once a year or so. Ultimately, your personal preferences for your appearance will determine the goals of these types of treatments.

Dermal fillers are injected directly into the middle skin layer – called the dermis – or sometimes into deeper areas. These treatments can be especially effective in correcting or improving the appearance of sagging facial contours.

The most popular types of dermal fillers are:

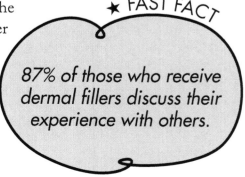

★ FAST FACT

87% of those who receive dermal fillers discuss their experience with others.

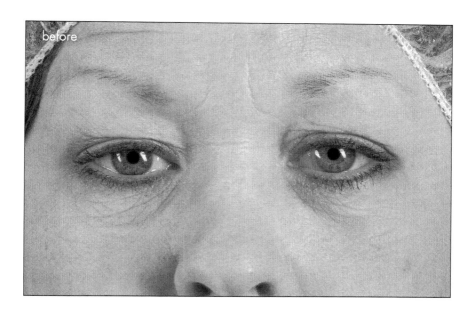

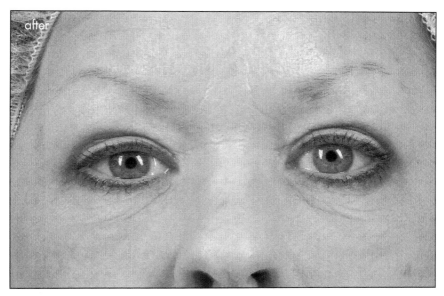

As a heavy smoker, this patient's skin had developed many deep lines. After BOTOX®, laser resurfacing, filler to her lips, and an upper eyelid lift, she appears more alert and refreshed.

★ **Collagen,** which is found in the body's bone, skin, cartilage, and tendons, is a natural protein that gives skin strength and elasticity. It can also be effective in filling in facial lines.

★ **Restylane™, JUVEDERM®, Perlane™,** which are all made from hyaluronic acid, are extremely safe and generally used around the cheeks, mouth area, the eyes, and for lip augmentation.

★ **Sculptra™ (poly-L-lactic acid),** which stimulates the growth of collagen, is especially effective in treating fat loss under the skin's surface. It tends to work best on sunken cheeks, which can also contribute to an aged, tired looking face.

★ **Radiesse™,** which consists of small beads of calcium, almost like a bone paste, is a semi-permanent filler. It is thicker and it lasts longer than the other fillers.

Biocompatible injectable fillers will fill out hollow areas and create a more youthful and aesthetically pleasing curvature that extends from the eyelid to the cheekbones, creating a smooth appearance, firming the appearance of lower eyelids, and effectively eliminating dark circles under the eyes.

The most popular wrinkle smoothers used around the eyes are BOTOX® and Dysport®. These are both forms of botulinum toxin type A, a purified protein that relaxes muscle contraction and smoothes the wrinkles that form with repeated frowning expressions.

Will my eye treatment hurt?

Typically, injections are painless enough that no anesthesia is necessary, but a local anesthetic may be given to make you as comfortable as possible. Another option is a topical or cream anesthetic, which numbs the injection site so you won't feel any pain or soreness during your treatment.

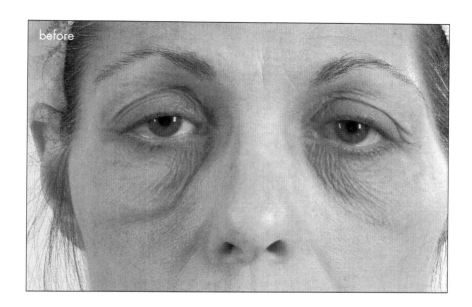

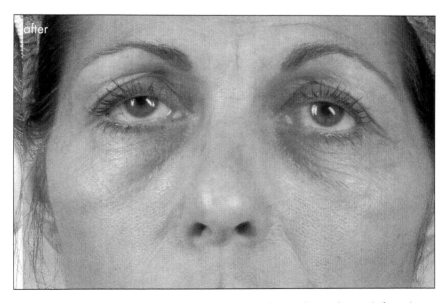

This patient lost a considerable amount of weight and was left with sagging skin and facial wrinkles around her eyes. She had BOTOX®, fillers, and laser resurfacing to appear more alert.

In most cases, patients are surprised by the minimal discomfort that they feel from their injection treatment. The vast majority of people are able to return to their normal activities, including work and exercise, immediately after their procedure. Some people do experience mild tenderness in the treated area, but nothing significant enough to interfere with your normal routine.

> ★ FAST FACT
>
> Restylane™, JUVEDERM®, and Hylaform™ dermal fillers were used in over 1.25 million treatments in 2008.

The simple procedure of injecting fillers into your eye area usually only takes between five and fifteen minutes, which means you can have your treatment during a lunch hour and be back at work right away. For most individuals, side effects may sometimes include very mild bruising, redness, swelling, or tenderness at your injection sites. Risk of allergic reactions or infections is unlikely, making this a safe, effective treatment for almost anyone. On occasion bruising can be more noticeable after this treatment, although this can vary.

What about after my treatment?

Any swelling or puffiness you experience post-treatment may last for one to two weeks. Cold compresses and over-the-counter pain medication can reduce any discomfort you feel. Usually these symptoms disappear quickly, although your diet as well as individual physiological factors will affect how you personally recover from your treatment.

Keep in mind that swelling after a filler injection is completely normal. Fillers usually attract water to the area of injection, which contributes to swelling. Often this swelling is insignificant enough that people around you won't notice it. You, on the other hand, are more likely to be aware of it because you are most familiar with your own face and you may feel a puffy

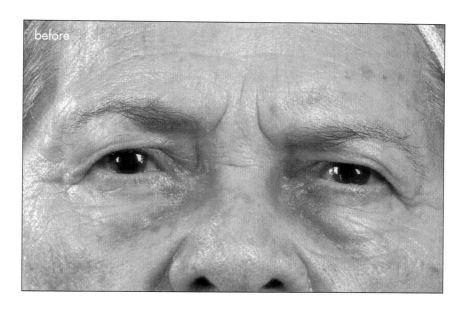

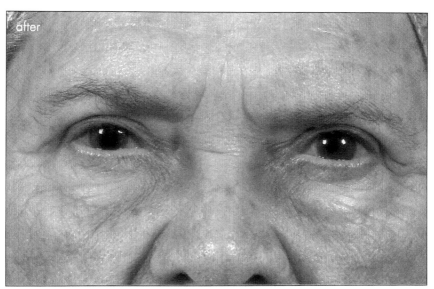

After removing the heavy skin from the upper lids, this patient appears less tired and more alert.

sensation in the treated area.

Bruising is not common, but it can occur. This is completely normal and noticeable bruising should disappear within one week, although it can take longer in rarer instances.

Because eyelid skin is so thin, even very mild bruising can be quite apparent. This is completely normal and noticeable bruising should disappear within one week. Your tendency to bruise will play a big factor in whether you bruise at all, how noticeable your bruises will be, and how long they will last.

Injection treatments are relatively straightforward procedures, which means you won't need any stitches or bandages. This can make you a lot more comfortable interacting with your family or people at work immediately after your treatment. Because these procedures only involve pinpoint-sized injections, scarring is not a typical risk.

What will I look like when it's all done?

The type of treatment you choose will affect how long it takes for your results to be completely apparent. BOTOX® takes about a week to achieve its full effect, which means you will have to be patient while your new look gradually reveals itself. With fillers, the results are immediate. You should see your new, desirable look in the mirror as soon as the treatment is over.

The type of filler as well as the size of the treatment area will affect the longevity of your treatment. Many treatments have virtually permanent results, while others can last around six months or more. Depending on what you are hoping to achieve and what the initial condition of your eye area is, some dermal fillers will not be permanent solutions, but may need to be performed on a yearly basis.

Fat transfers, on the other hand, tend to be permanent, but in some cases a repeat procedure may be necessary to generate the desired result. You should discuss your ultimate goals for your treatment with your doctor so that he is clear on what you want to achieve. Your doctor can give you a

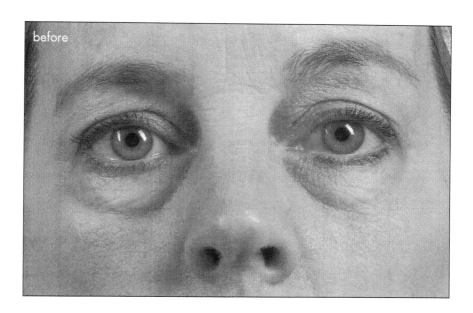

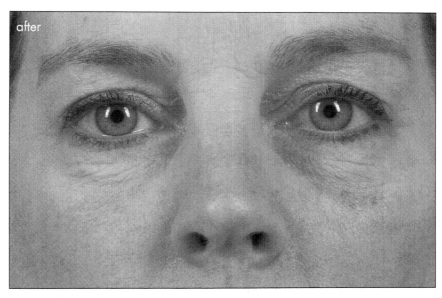

Filler placed into the hollows under the eyes and into the cheeks results in a more youthful, relaxed look with outstanding improvement of lower eyelid bags without surgery.

general timeframe for the duration of your results and advise you of any maintenance treatment routines that may be necessary.

Patients who undergo injectable filler procedures achieve a youthful and fresh appearance to the area around and below the eyelids. The area under the eyes loses that sagging, tired look. Dark circles and hollows can virtually disappear with as few as one treatment. Because these procedures have no downtime, you can literally replace your tired eyes with younger, fresher and more alert ones in only about ten minutes.

These treatments can be a simple solution to the bothersome problem of tired looking eyes. Talk to your doctor about your options so that you can once again have the energetic, youthful eyes you deserve.

★ FAST FACT

There were more than 58,000 treatments using collagen in 2008.

Q & A WITH DR. KOTLUS.

Q **How long will the effects of my procedure last? Will I need to have repeat procedures?**

A That depends on exactly what is being performed and the person's natural response to that procedure. So there's no simple answer, but there's a range of timeframes are possible. A procedure such as BOTOX® may last four to five months, fillers may last eight to nine months, a laser may last for several years, and a combination of these things can last anywhere over that entire timeframe.

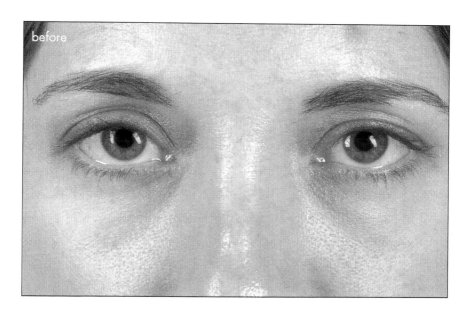

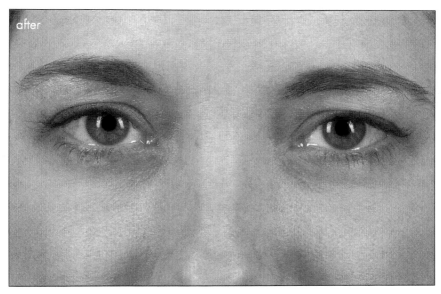

Injectable filler placed in the area between the lower eyelids and cheeks eliminates hollowing and shadowing associated with "looking tired."

✔ CHECKLIST

☐ What kind of dermal filler is best for me and my skin type?

_____

_____

_____

_____

☐ Would I be better off with a fat transfer? Which procedure will offer better results?

_____

_____

_____

_____

☐ If I have the fat injections, what will happen if I gain or lose weight?

_____

_____

_____

_____

☐ Will I be awake or asleep during the procedure?

_____

_____

_____

_____

☐ Is the procedure painful? Will I be uncomfortable after the process?

_____

_____

_____

_____

☐ What will I look like when the procedure is finished?

_____

_____

_____

_____

☐ Will I have any scars?

_____

_____

_____

_____

_____

☐ Are there any risks or complications with a fat injection or dermal filler injection procedure?

_____

_____

_____

_____

_____

QUICK QUESTIONS: *Looking Tired*

Is there anesthesia?

There is typically no anesthesia. Occasionally a local or topical cream anesthetic can be used.

Where would the procedure take place?

The procedure usually takes place in a doctor's office.

How long will the procedure take to complete?

The procedure will take five to fifteen minutes to complete.

What is the level of discomfort I should expect?

Discomfort is usually minimal during and after the procedure.

Will there be bruising?

Usually there's no bruising, but occasionally it can happen, especially with a person taking aspirin, vitamin E or fish oil.

Will there be any swelling?

For the first day or so fillers can attract water and result in some swelling. Usually it is something the patient would notice, but wouldn't be enough for other people notice. This obviously varies.

Will there be any numbness?

Numbness is not commonly an issue with this procedure.

What type of bandages will I wear and when do the bandages come off?

There are no bandages for this procedure.

Are there any stitches?

There are no stitches used.

When can I go back to work?

Some people go back to work the same day.

When can I start exercising again?

You can resume exercise the same day in most cases.

When can I expect the final result?

For BOTOX®, it will take a week or so to get the full result. With a dermal filler, the result is apparent right away.

★ NOTES

★ NOTES

Chapter 7 ★

Help For Unsightly Veins

★ CHAPTER HIGHLIGHTS:

★ Veins are a crucial part of the body, taking blood back to the heart to be oxygenated and pushed back into the body via the arteries.

★ Genetics can play a role in the development of unsightly veins.

★ Varicose veins are the larger and bulging veins, while spider veins are much smaller and more of a cosmetic problem than uncomfortable.

★ Bulging veins can be painful and cause feelings of heaviness, itchiness, or restlessness.

★ Over time, veins become less effective and can have valve leaks, which enlarges the veins and causes them to bulge.

★ Varicose veins and spider veins can be treated separately, but as varicose veins feed the spider veins, it's best to treat the larger veins first.

★ The procedures are nearly painless and patients are back up on their feet immediately.

Can I get help for these unattractive veins?

If you're one of the many who avoid wearing shorts in the summertime because of your veins, you'll be happy to learn that today there are numerous options to help you reveal nicer looking legs with confidence.

Not only are your visible veins unattractive, but they can also mean pain and swelling, especially during warmer weather and physical activity. These veins – known as spider veins or varicose veins – are usually on your legs, but they can be found in other areas of the body, too. Some people complain of veins on their noses, chests, hands, or under their eyes. Since these spots are usually visible to the outside world, it's no wonder you want to get rid of them.

Your veins are responsible for carrying your blood back to your lungs so that it can be reoxygenated, and it's not an easy job. This is an endless task that is in progress every day of your life, which means your veins are constantly working to make sure your blood has the oxygen it needs to make your body run.

Your veins have one-way valves in them to keep your blood moving in the proper direction, but over time, these valves can stop working as well as they should. Your veins also tend to get a little larger with age, and the combination of these two things can make your veins more prone to protruding to the point of being visible under your skin's surface.

This process can also cause pressure to build up in your veins, which is likely the root of any pain you're experiencing in and around those unsightly veins. Over time, the pressure can actually create sores on your skin's surface. Some people also report feelings of heaviness or fatigue in their legs, itching, and even occasionally restless leg symptoms.

The good news is that this is all happening in your

★ FAST FACT

Of all non-surgical cosmetic procedures performed in 2007, almost 2% were either sclerotherapy or laser treatments for leg veins.

superficial veins only, which means it's likely not dangerous (i.e. you don't have to worry about blood clots). You'll also be pleased to know that these conditions are treatable and, in many cases, your doctor can make your unsightly veins seem to disappear.

★ FAST FACT

In 2007, sclerotherapy was the 8th most common non-surgical cosmetic procedure for females, while being the 25th most common for males.

What are my options?

The old method of getting rid of unsightly veins was to do something called vein stripping, which could be quite painful, had a long downtime associated with it, and almost always had to be repeated.

Today, cosmetic surgeons can offer you quicker, virtually painless, and relatively permanent options to deal with your veins. The two main types of unattractive veins, spider veins and varicose veins, each have modern treatments designed to minimize their appearance.

Spider veins

Spider veins are the smaller of the two visible vein types. These can be quite hard to see on most people, although just knowing they're there can hamper your self-confidence. Spider veins won't normally cause you pain, but they can definitely make you feel less than presentable in shorts or a skirt.

For these types of visible veins, sclerotherapy is the current standard of care. During this procedure, you simply get small injections of a sclerosing agent, which essentially closes up your spider veins, making them virtually invisible.

In some cases, your cosmetic surgeon will opt for foam injections to help minimize the appearance of your spider veins. Lasers have proven effective in

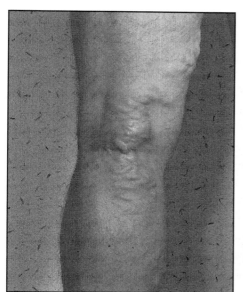
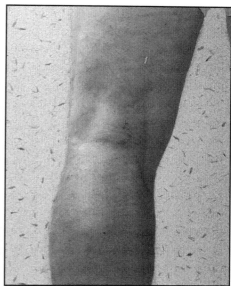

Before receiving treatment (left), patient had bulging varicose veins. Six weeks after treatment (right), veins have begun to break down and will continue to disappear over a couple of months.

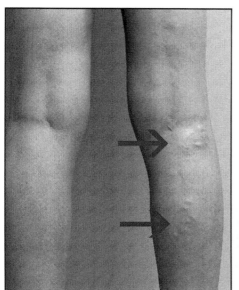
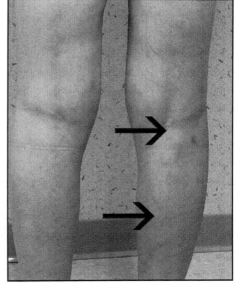

Patient has visible varicose veins before treatment (left). After treatment (right), veins have begun to disappear. This patient will continue to see improvement before seeing the final result in a couple of months.

certain cases, as well. Your doctor will let you know which type of treatment will work best in your particular circumstance. Both lasers and foam work to irritate the veins in question, causing them to close and shrink so they are not visible.

Varicose veins

Varicose veins are significantly bigger than spider veins, which means they are more visible and often seem to bulge out of your skin. This bulging can be very uncomfortable and can also cause discomfort in the surrounding skin. If you have pain associated with your unsightly veins, you can bet that varicose veins are to blame.

The current and most effective varicose vein treatment involves lasers. Called "endovenous laser ablation," this process uses a very small laser fiber inserted into the offending vein. The energy from the laser causes the vein to start closing up, which reduces its size and bulge, as well as any associated pain. Another treatment called radiofrequency vein ablation works in the same way, but uses radiofrequency energy to close the veins instead of a laser. Both are effective.

Sometimes, your varicose veins will "feed" your smaller veins and cause them to become visible in some cases. Dealing with your varicose veins can therefore have the added benefit of reducing your spider veins as well.

Which procedure is best for me?

Your doctor can help you decide what type of treatment is ideal to minimize the look of your unattractive veins. You may have the option of just treating either your spider veins or your varicose veins. In many cases, however, the best way to improve the look of your legs or other troubled areas will be to have a

★ FAST FACT

After a vein treatment, patients are able to immediately return to work- there's no downtime!

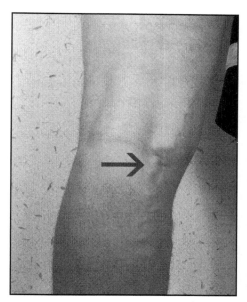 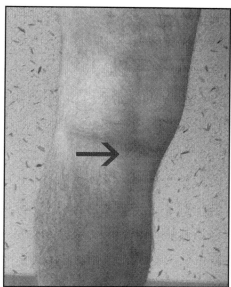

Pronounced varicose veins (left) have nearly disappeared
two months after treatment (right).

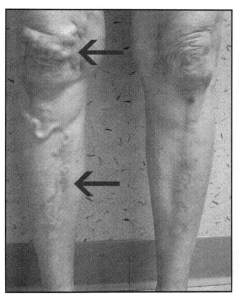 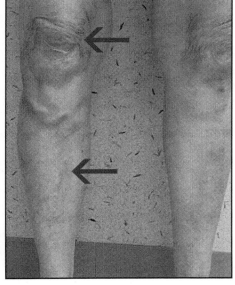

Patient has noticeable varicose veins (left). Seven days after receiving just a single
non-surgical vein treatment, this patient has already seen a great reduction in the
appearance of veins. Veins will continue to dissipate and break down over the next
two months, so she can expect to see a continued improvement in their appearance.

combination of procedures performed. Usually, this means a mixture of both laser treatments and sclerotherapy.

Will my procedure(s) hurt?

While your unsightly veins themselves may cause you pain, the treatments to deal with them are thankfully relatively painless.

With laser treatments, you will feel a degree of pain as the laser is directed into the vein, but the feeling is minor and the procedure itself is over quickly. Your personal pain threshold will be a factor in how much pain you actually feel.

With sclerotherapy, the injections are performed with very small needles, so you will have very little pain – if any – while your procedure is taking place. If you are sensitive, you may feel a slight pinch at the injection site; otherwise, you may not feel anything.

What about after my procedure?

Because these procedures are relatively minor, you shouldn't have any downtime at all. In fact, your cosmetic surgeon will encourage you to be up on your feet as quickly as possible after your procedure. This is because sitting can cause your blood to repool, which may reduce or undo the results produced by your treatments.

You may experience a small amount of soreness post-treatment, but this can easily be subdued with over-the-counter pain medications in most cases. Any pain you do experience should dissipate within a day or so.

You may also notice slight brown patches around your treatment areas after your procedure. These patches are actually blood that has repooled, but over time – up to a year – they tend to disappear. Remember to get up and move around as soon as possible after your treatment to minimize the appearance of these patches. Your doctor may also be able to treat any spots you aren't happy

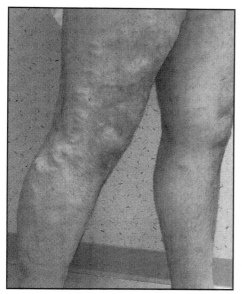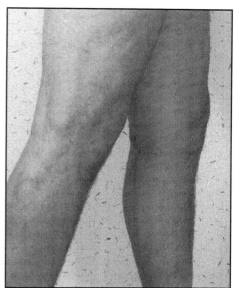

Patient with bulging varicose veins before treatment (left) and one week after treatment (right). The appearance of veins will continue to improve over the next one to two months.

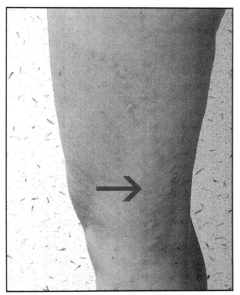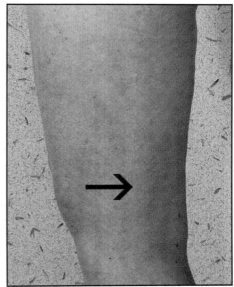

This patient received non-surgical treatment for her pronounced varicose veins as well as Mesotherapy for cellulite and fat.

with to make them dissipate more quickly.

Rarely can the brown spots last longer than six months. Other uncommon risks include skin sores. Wearing compression stockings as directed after the procedure will help to prevent certain problems including blood clots. Your doctor will monitor for these and explain how they are treated if they occur.

What am I going to look like when it's all done?

Your spider and varicose veins – even the biggest, most bothersome ones – will likely completely vanish after your cosmetic procedure.

If your varicose veins were particularly troublesome, any pain they were causing you will likely disappear. That means that you can enjoy warmer weather and physical activity without the pain associated with your previously bulging veins.

Unfortunately, it is possible for your unsightly veins to return. This is especially true for those small spider veins, although just how long your treatment will last will be affected both by your lifestyle and your genes.

If you're on your feet a lot, you are putting more strain on your veins. That means that people like teachers and nurses will probably see a quicker resurgence of their unsightly veins than people with other kinds of jobs.

Your genetic makeup will also play a role in how long your treatments last. If your parents have had trouble with spider and varicose veins, there's an increased chance that you will too. Your treatments – especially for your spider veins – may need to be repeated at regular intervals, especially if your veins were stubborn during initial treatments. Your doctor can help you determine what kind of treatment schedule you might expect.

★ FAST FACT

Unlike vein stripping, new vein treatment technologies are minimally invasive and nearly painless.

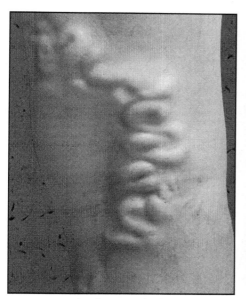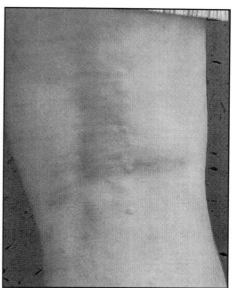

Patient had severe bulging veins. Six months after treatment, the treated
veins have disappeared.

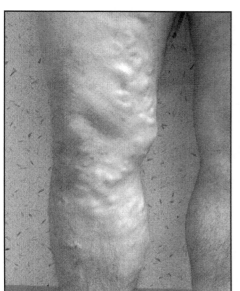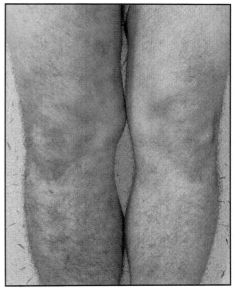

This patient had severe varicose veins. Four months after treatment,
appearance is much improved and veins are no longer visible.

If you are concerned you might be putting excessive strain on your veins, consider purchasing knee-high compression stockings. These stockings help your blood continue to flow in the proper direction, which reduces pooling caused by leaky valves. You may find them especially helpful if your job has you on your feet for extended periods of time or if you think you have an unfortunate combination of genes.

★ FAST FACT

Varicose and spider veins are not deep veins. They are only found in the superficial layers of the skin.

Of course, most people who treat their spider and varicose veins also experience a surge in self-esteem, especially during the warmer months. These treatments truly are a simple way to get rid of veins that have made you self-conscious about your appearance.

Q & A WITH DR. KOTLUS.

Q **Will my skin be changed or lightened by the laser treatments?**

A Your skin will not be lightened by the procedure, but one of the after-effects that you could actually get are brown spots that look like bruising. These are usually the result of blood that's trapped within the treated vein, and it takes the body time to get rid of that trapped blood. During that time, there could be a brown patch, which can actually look like a stain in the skin, that consists of iron that's found in the blood. There are cases where it could take six months to a year for this to stop. Any skin change tends to related to this sort of discoloration.

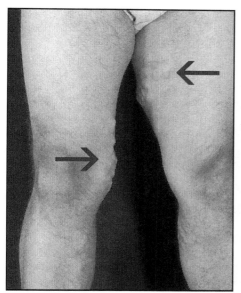
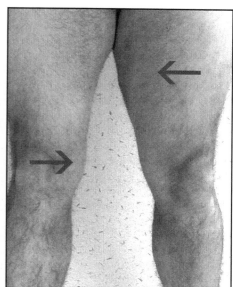

This patient received laser ablation and micro foam injections for his varicose veins. The photo on the right was taken six months after treatment.

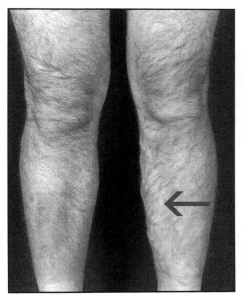
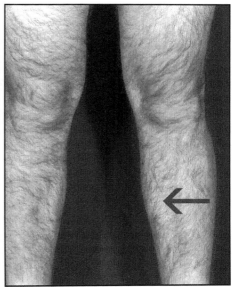

This patient had noticeable varicose veins. Seven months after non-surgical vein treatment, the appearance of the veins is greatly improved.

★ TREATING HER VARICOSE VEINS HELPED ONE WOMAN TO JUMP-START HER NEW, HEALTHIER LIFESTYLE!

Renata, 59 years-old, has suffered from painful varicose veins for over twenty years. She has undergone various treatments to combat the unsightly veins, including vein stripping.

Last spring, a local radio station hosted an open house at Allure Medical Spa. So I went, being a person who has suffered from varicose veins since my mid 30's. I was really interested and asked a lot of questions. There were other patients who you could talk to, which I think is the best thing for a person deciding whether or not to have a procedure. And they did a presentation, answered questions, and by the end of the night I signed up for an exam.

I inherited varicose veins from both sides of my family, and I used to work as a floral designer so I stood on a rubber mat on a cement floor for years. I am a little overweight, which doesn't cause varicose veins but it probably doesn't help, but it nice to find out that heredity is the biggest factor, along with your job. Nurses, teachers, anybody standing on their feet all day is more likely to develop varicose veins. So I was relieved to find out that it wasn't anything that I did to myself. Starting in my 30's, I had swelling in the legs, soreness, and achiness, and I was more concerned about my looks then too. Varicose veins are pretty unsightly, they're blue, they're like a road map on your legs. But the reason I went to the doctor in the first place was the pain, the ache and the swelling. I had vein stripping in 1990 and I had saline injection in 1999. The vein stripping treatments helped for a while, but that means you have to go in to the hospital, you have general anesthesia, you're out of work and have to be home for a few days.

The exam was very, very thorough, I think I was there for a couple of hours. I went in there with a lot of questions. The first thing I think that everybody's afraid of is pain. Is this gonna hurt me? And they talked about the 2 different procedures, one was the laser and one was what they call "foam" - it's an injection. My big question about the foam was, is anybody allergic to it? There will be a rare case when someone is, and what if I'm that rare case, what can you do about it? It was very comforting to know that they're prepared to handle any emergency, if indeed you were allergic to it. I was not and it was wonderful. I had both the laser and the injections, but I really don't have a preference. I think the injections were quicker, if you can take a mosquito bite, you're fine. It's not pain- I can't stress that enough for people when they ask, does it hurt? No! And the laser, they numb your leg up, you'll just feel a pinch, that's it! So there isn't any pain, and I also wondered, am I going to bleed? What will happen? But it's no worse that taking a blood test. So those were my biggest concerns: pain, bleeding, or a reaction, and I had none of those.

When I went in there for the first procedure, I cried. I was so embarrassed about my legs. They were really unsightly. All these green veins, it's not pretty. The staff made me feel so comfortable, they're wonderful, and they share their own stories from different procedures. They were so open that you leave there hugging people, it's really how they are. My daughter came with me to every procedure. They encouraged her questions; they let her come in to the room. They explained everything – every step of the way. So, I can't say enough about their staff, they're just wonderful. And another thing is that I don't have to miss work. I came back to work the same day. There's really no down time here. You're there for a little while, then you walk for 20 minutes, then you go back to work

That's the one thing that you have to do after every procedure: walk. You walk for 20 minutes to keep your circulation going . Well, the walking has become a habit for me and a plus is I've lost 30 pounds! I've continued the walking and they are so supportive. For me, this has become a health issue. My husband passed away at 53 from cancer.

I don't want my kids to lose another parent. I'm to the point now where I feel like I have to "step up to the plate." So this walking has been great - my cardiologist is happy, I am happy, Dr. Mok is happy, and I'm telling you my legs feel great! I just went to Belle Isle for the cancer walk on Saturday, and I didn't do 5 miles, but I sure went farther than in the last two years. So I can not say enough about these people and these procedures. I'm happy, my legs are happy, my kids are happy. Because you can get down, you know? You get all these medical issues, but I can't do anything about yesterday. I can't. What I can do is do something about today, and tomorrow, and I'll tell you, Allure Medical Spa was my jump-start. And I just wish I had done this a few years ago, you know. I'm so happy with them.

And you know what? I don't have to guard my legs anymore. Anytime I went anywhere where you're sitting at a table with people, I would guard my legs so that no one would bump them, because I was afraid of bumping the veins. So I no longer have to make sure that my legs are guarded. I look down, I still have weight to lose, I still have heavier legs than I what I would like, but I do not see those blue ridges, those mountains, the topographical map on my legs. It makes me so happy that I could wear a dress if I wanted to. I can't say enough about them and their procedures and their staff. I can't recommend them enough!

✔ CHECKLIST

☐ Am I good candidate for vein treatments?

_____

_____

_____

_____

☐ What are the differences between laser vein treatments and sclerotherapy? Which is the best treatment for me?

_____

_____

_____

_____

☐ Do I need to prepare my skin in any way before the procedure?

_____

_____

_____

_____

☐ What are the side effects I can expect? What should I do about them?

_____

_____

_____

_____

☐ What are the risks of this vein treatment?

_____

_____

_____

_____

☐ How can I maintain my vein treatment
results after the treatment?

_____

_____

_____

_____

☐ How much pain can I expect during and
after the vein treatment?

_____

_____

_____

_____

☐ What happens if I have an allergic
reaction to the treatment?

_____

_____

_____

_____

QUICK
QUESTIONS: *Unsightly Veins*

Is there anesthesia?

There is local anesthesia.

Where would the procedure take place?

The procedure takes place in an office or in an office-like setting (at the hospital).

How long will the procedure take to complete?

There is usually a series of procedures to deal with veins, but the individual sessions usually last from fifteen to thirty minutes.

What is the level of discomfort I should expect?

The discomfort is minimal for most patients. Patients say the sensation is equivalent to having blood drawn.

Will there be bruising?

About half of patients get bruising, which can take a week or two to go down, sometimes even a few weeks.

Will there be any swelling?

Swelling tends to be variable.

Will there be any numbness?

Numbness is rare, but can happen. See your doctor if there is any prolonged numbness.

What type of bandages will I wear and when do the bandages come off?

You'll wear a compression stocking for 2 days after each procedure is performed.

Are there any stitches?

No.

When can I go back to work?

You can go back to work immediately.

When can I start exercising again?

You can go exercise immediately.

When can I expect the final result?

You'll see everything completely healed within a few months.

★ NOTES

★ NOTES

Chapter 8 ★

Tummy Tucks Explained

★ CHAPTER HIGHLIGHTS:

★ A tummy tuck may be the perfect solution to a sagging waistline created by pregnancy, weight loss, aging, or genetics.

★ There are two types of tummy tuck: one that removes extra skin alone and one that combines liposuction with skin removal.

★ You may also have your tummy muscles tightened during your tummy tuck to create a stronger-looking, flatter stomach.

★ All tummy tucks are designed to give you a permanently smooth tummy and a slimmer waistline.

★ Your tummy tuck will be performed under anesthesia.

★ Your doctor will prescribe pain medication to alleviate any discomfort you feel after the surgery.

What can a tummy tuck do for me?

Being a woman has its share of blessings. Pregnancy and motherhood, though difficult, are two beautiful aspects of life that men can never know.

Of course, in addition to being busy mothers, wives, and/or career professionals, women also like to feel like women: beautiful, energetic, and vibrant.

★ FAST FACT

The number of tummy tucks performed in North America has increased by about 445% in the last thirteen years.

A sagging tummy that results from pregnancy, aging, or dramatic weight loss can certainly be a little…well, depressing. This physical change is often an unavoidable side effect of enjoying your life as a woman. It can be especially disheartening to have an unattractive, always-there bulge when you've worked so hard to create a family or shed those extra pounds.

Although your skin is extremely elastic and resilient, if it stretches past a certain point it simply can't bounce back on its own. Think of a metal spring: you can pull on it and it will spring right back into place, but if you pull too far, the connections between the actual metal atoms will change and the spring just won't be able to regain its original shape. A similar principle exists with the skin around your midsection.

★ FAST FACT

Modern tummy tucks can be combined with liposuction to produce dramatic changes in your waistline and overall appearance.

A tummy tuck may be the solution to do away with extra skin or stubborn fat deposits for good. There are a couple of procedures you can choose from and both can help you create the flattering body shape that you deserve.

What are my options?

There are two major types of abdominoplasty – or tummy tucks – and the amount of fat you have around your midsection will play a part in determining which one is best for you. You should discuss your ideal body shape with your doctor beforehand so he understands your goals and desired outcome.

Traditional tummy tucks

The traditional tummy tuck involves making an incision to create a flap under your skin and abdominal fat. Your surgeon pulls this flap down and removes any excess at the bottom. The incision is then closed and the result is a smoother, flatter stomach.

If you have a larger area of hanging skin, your belly button may be relocated to a new position during your procedure. This is done when your tummy tuck would result in your belly button being either in an unnatural-looking position or would actually be removed if it remained in its original place. Relocating your belly button to a more appropriate position will help make your tummy tuck look as natural as possible.

Combitucks™

A newer procedure, called the Combituck™ (also termed Avelar abdominoplasty or lipo-abdominoplasty), involves some liposuction in addition to your tummy tuck. A Combituck™ can be the perfect option if you've got unwanted fat in the area in addition to the extra skin. Along with removing any hanging, bulging skin, your doctor will also literally

★ FAST FACT

Your favorite jeans or even a bikini will often hide a tummy tuck scar!

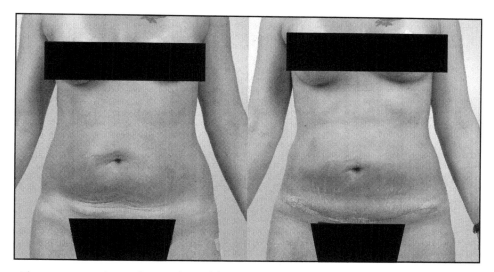

This patient, who is the mother of four children, had a Combituck and a breast lift with augmentation. The photo on the right was taken one week after her procedures. Although there can be some swelling and bruising with these procedures, it is usually minimal.

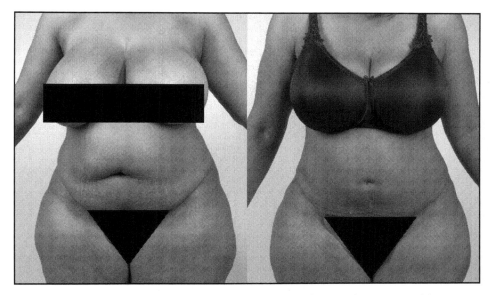

This 33 year-old patient's husband is in the military. She surprised him while he was away with a Combituck, which improves the loose skin of the midsection while removing extra fat.

suction out any stubborn fat that has been lingering around your midsection.

Not surprisingly, this procedure can produce a gorgeous figure. You and your doctor can discuss how much extra fat you have in your tummy area and how much you'd like to get rid of during your tummy tuck.

★ FAST FACT

Tummy tucks are one of the top five most common surgical procedures performed by cosmetic surgeons across North America.

As with the traditional tummy tuck, your Combituck™ may include the relocation of your belly button. Your doctor can show you where your belly button would end up with or without relocation so you can get an idea of what will look best on you.

Important information about your tummy tuck

Whichever procedure you have, your surgeon may also want to tighten up any loose abdominal muscles you may have acquired over the years. Loose tummy muscles are common in aging women or women who have been pregnant or have lost a lot of weight. This is because abdominal stretching, the passage of time, or even a genetic predisposition can cause your tummy muscles to separate and lose their strength. Like your skin, your muscles can only stretch so far before they won't rebound on their own.

Your procedure will likely take between two and five hours, depending on which type of tummy tuck you're having, how much fat is removed, and whether your abdominal muscles require tightening. Both types of tummy tucks involve an incision that will be carefully sutured closed at the end of your procedure.

The results of either tummy tuck procedure are virtually permanent, but be aware that if you get pregnant or gain a lot of weight after your tummy tuck, your results will more than likely change. Pregnancy and weight

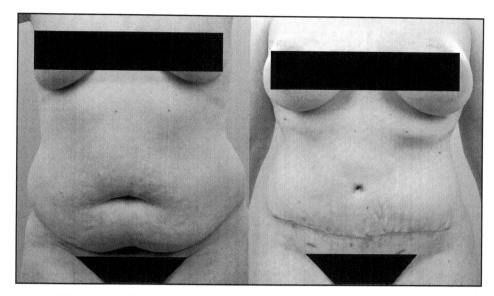

This patient had a breast augmentation and Combituck performed together. This procedure removed most of her stretch marks. The ones that are remaining look better when the skin is tighter.

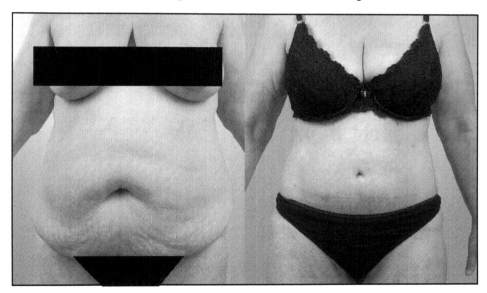

A combituck procedure removed the skin apron and shaped her torso. This motivated her to continue losing weight, and she had to replace her wardrobe because her old clothes no longer fit.

gain are two issues that can seriously undermine the longevity of your new, flatter tummy. Speak to your doctor about any potential body changes you may be anticipating down the road. Your doctor may recommend postponing your tummy tuck until you're done having children or give you helpful advice about staying trim through healthy eating and exercise.

★ FAST FACT

People between the ages of 35 and 64 make up over 76% of tummy tuck patients. Over 97% of those patients are women.

Will my tummy tuck hurt?

Both types of tummy tucks are done under anesthesia, which means you are not fully conscious. Traditional tummy tucks are performed under general anesthesia. In these cases, you are totally asleep during the procedure.

For the Combituck™, you may be a candidate for local anesthetic, plus a sedative. Many patients opt for this because sedatives can involve less time to "come out of" than general anesthetic, while the actual effects during your procedure are identical to those of general anesthetic – no memory of the actual procedure.

Whichever anesthetic you choose, trained specialists will monitor you before, during, and after your tummy tuck. Your doctor can discuss which options are best for you.

What about after my tummy tuck?

You will probably experience some discomfort after your tummy tuck, although just how much will depend on the type of procedure you have as well as your personal tolerance for pain.

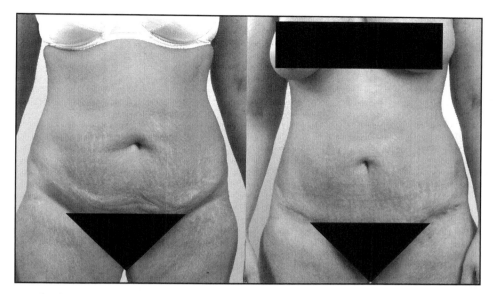

The loose skin on the lower belly was tightened with a mini combituck. the incision line will fade over time and become less red. this photo was taken 1 month after surgery.

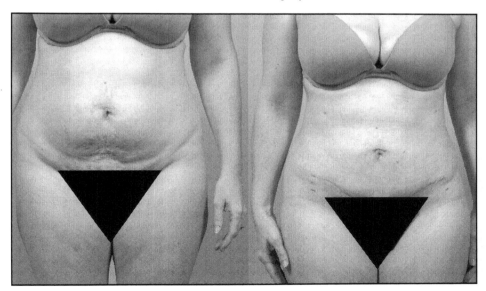

before and after mini combituck, resulting in a nicer shape and tighter skin of the lower belly.

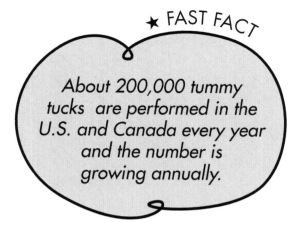

★ FAST FACT

About 200,000 tummy tucks are performed in the U.S. and Canada every year and the number is growing annually.

The Combituck™ – the tummy tuck plus some liposuction – is actually less involved surgically than the traditional tummy tuck. This means that you should expect only about a week of tenderness after the procedure. This option helps you get back to your everyday life relatively quickly.

The traditional tummy tuck, on the other hand, involves several weeks of tenderness and general downtime from the more strenuous aspects of your day-to-day life. You should plan to take two to four weeks off from work and physical activity.

With both procedures, you will also experience some swelling around the surgical area. This is perfectly normal. When your body experiences an incision, swelling occurs both to help close the opening and to provide the fluids necessary to heal the area.

Whichever tummy tuck is right for you, you should know that the downtime after your procedure doesn't mean you'll be confined to bed or in constant pain. Discomfort is normal, but your doctor will prescribe medication so you can control pain you may feel. You will certainly be able to walk around and do light activity. Only strenuous activity, such as heavy lifting, sit-ups, or sports will have to be avoided. Your cosmetic surgeon can tell you exactly which activities you should stay away from and for how long.

What am I going to look like when it's all done?

Women who are tummy tuck candidates are understandably disheartened by their belly bulge, especially when it's on the heels of something as fulfilling as pregnancy or dramatic weight loss.

It's very common for women to worry about scarring as a result of their tummy tuck. Because the procedure does involve an incision, you should expect some scarring. In many cases, the incision will be well below your waistline, so your scar will be all but unnoticeable except when you're totally nude. In other words, the scar can usually be hidden when wearing pants and even a bathing suit. You should ask your surgeon about your options for incision placement as well as what you can do to minimize scarring.

If you've had a cesarean section in the past, you'll be pleased to know that your doctor can likely use the same incision to perform your tummy tuck. Often the incision required for your tummy tuck is longer than what you needed for your cesarean delivery, but otherwise it can usually be placed in the same location on your abdomen.

Again, do your best to maintain your new waistline by eating well and exercising regularly. Your doctor can give you advice on staying trim so that you can enjoy your new, shapelier figure for the years and decades to come.

Q & A WITH DR. KOTLUS.

Q **What will happen if I gain or lose weight after my tummy tuck?**

A Losing weight after a tummy tuck usually enhances the result. Gaining a lot of weight is not suggested, but it can happen. If fat collects in your abdomen again the skin can stretch. Ultimately the goal would be to maintain weight or even reduce it somewhat.

★ HOW A BUSY MOTHER OF TWO GOT RID OF HER "MOM POUCH" AND BACK TO A FLAT STOMACH!

Katie is a twenty-nine-year-old mother of two. She works as an ultrasound technician, and has worked with thousands of women who have had cosmetic surgery. Last year she decided that it was time for her to fix something that had been bothering her: a sagging tummy.

I have two children, a nine-year-old and a five-year-old, and I delivered both through c-section. Afterward, I had a flap of skin with fat in it that, no matter how much dieting and exercise I did, it never went away. I hated the way it looked in jeans and I wanted it gone.

I really didn't have any concerns before the procedure, because I've seen what good results people have after they have it done, and it's almost immediate. I think you definitely need to believe in what you do and everyday at work, you know, I see the results. I see how happy people are after they have it done. You have to have confidence in the people that you work for and I definitely have a lot of confidence in Dr. Mok and Dr. Kotlus. They have great results, and their patients are very happy when it's all done.

I had the procedure done on a Friday, after work. It only took a few hours and immediately you could see the results! After having two c-sections, I didn't think it would be that bad, and it wasn't. The next day my stomach was

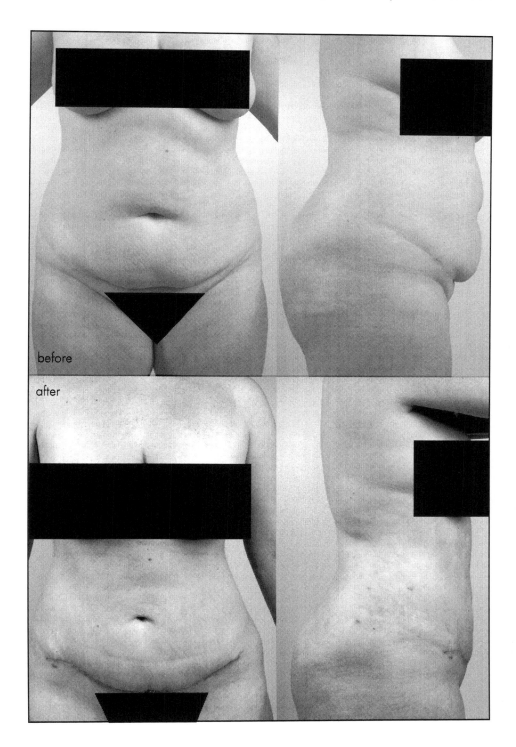

before

after

completely flat; you could see my muscles immediately. Saturday night my husband and I went to a party. I just had my bandage garment on under my blue jeans and no one knew I had anything done. I took it easy, but I could stand around and talk to people. I had very minimal swelling. I didn't have a whole lot of bruising and I was pretty much back to doing my normal activities by Monday. My husband went back to work and I had to take the kids to school. I was a little bit slower but it really wasn't that bad. I came back to work on Tuesday for a full 12-hour shift, and just had to make a few adjustments at work. Two weeks later was Thanksgiving, and I was good by then. Three weeks later, it was my cousin's wedding, and I did the alligator on the floor with my sisters. I was pretty good!

I have a lot of friends now who are interested in having a tummy tuck. They're all having babies now and they have, you know, the little mom pouch, some more than others. So they're definitely interested in it, and you're not out of commission for days- being a busy mom, there is no way I could have done it if I was. Even my mom, who took me for my post-op the day after my procedure, wants to have it done! Her stomach is very similar to how mine was. She was wowed by it!

✔ CHECKLIST

☐ What kind of tummy tuck is best for me?

_____
_____
_____
_____

☐ Do my stomach muscles need tightening?

_____
_____
_____
_____
_____

☐ What are my options for anesthesia?

_____
_____
_____
_____

☐ How much discomfort can I expect after the surgery? For how long?

_____
_____
_____
_____
_____

☐ How long until I can go back to work or resume exercise?

_____

_____

_____

_____

☐ What will my waistline look like?

_____

_____

_____

_____

☐ Where will the incision be placed? Will it leave a noticeable scar?

_____

_____

_____

_____

☐ Is there a chance I will need a touch-up procedure sometime down the road?

_____

_____

_____

_____

QUICK QUESTIONS: *Tummy Tucks*

Is there anesthesia?

Yes, either general anesthesia or IV sedation with local anesthetic.

Where would the procedure take place?

The procedure takes place in an outpatient surgery center or hospital.

How long will the procedure take to complete?

The length of the procedure is approximately two to four hours. The total length of stay is between three and six hours.

What is the level of discomfort I should expect?

The discomfort is moderate. Usually the first week is the most sore period, but it will take a couple of weeks for that soreness to go away completely. You should avoid heavy activity for the first week or two, and it usually takes about three weeks until you're back to your normal routine.

Will there be bruising?

Bruising can be variable, usually for the first two weeks. After that it typically subsides.

Will there be any swelling?

It takes a couple of months before all the swelling goes down for most patients. The first two to three weeks the swelling will be the most noticeable.

Will there be any numbness?

There can be numbness around the incision area. That can last for a couple of weeks, or occasionally for a couple of months.

What type of bandages will I wear and when do the bandages come off?

You'll wear a compression garment for several weeks. And usually, on the incision there is a special type of dressing that comes off a week later.

Are there any stitches?

There are stitches, but they will dissolve inside, so there is no need to remove them.

When can I go back to work?

You can go back to work within two to three weeks.

When can I expect the final result?

Three to six months.

★ NOTES

★ NOTES

Glossary ★

ABCS: The American Board of Cosmetic Surgery, the only organization that solely certifies physicians in the practice of surgery to improve the appearance.

Abdominoplasty: A surgical procedure that flattens your abdomen by removing extra fat and skin, and tightening abdominal muscles. Commonly referred to as a tummy tuck.

Age spots: Flat pigmented spots seen on areas of the body exposed to the sun over time. Age spots usually occur after age 40.

Arnica: Also called Arnica Montana, this is a flowering herb used in homeopathic medicines designed to reduce bruising after surgery. There is little scientific evidence that Arnica is effective.

Blepharoplasty: A surgical procedure that reduces loose skin and/or fat from upper and/or lower eyelids. Sometimes combined with laser resurfacing and BOTOX®.

Breast augmentation: A surgical procedure done to increase breast size.

Body dysmorphic disorder: A psychological condition characterized by an excessive concern about a perceived physical defect.

BOTOX®: A purified protein (a form of botulinum toxin) that works by relaxing muscles that cause frowning. Also see Dysport

Brachioplasty: A surgical procedure also termed arm lift, which removes skin and/or fat to tighten and reshape the arm.

Brow lift: A surgical procedure in which the eyebrows are lifted to reduce droopiness above the eyes and forehead.

Chemical peel: A process in which a chemical solution is applied to the skin to remove surface skin cells and stimulate the production of new skin cells.

Collagen: The major structural protein in the skin that provides strength and tone.

Combituck: A form of tummy tuck that combines liposuction with the removal of loose skin. Also termed Avelar abdominoplasty or lipo-abdominoplasty.

Cosmetic surgeon: A doctor that performs surgical procedures to improve appearance. These surgeons may come from various backgrounds including dermatology, ear nose throat surgery, oculoplastic surgery, plastic surgery, and general surgery.

Crow's Feet: The radial smile lines found around the eyes.

Dermabrasion: A surgical procedure in which a patient's outer layers of skin are removed.

Dermis: The middle layer of the skin, composed of blood vessels, hair follicles, and oil glands. The dermis is where wrinkles occur.

Dysport: A form of botulinum toxin used to relax muscles that produce frown lines. Also see BOTOX®

Elastin: A protein found in the skin that contributes to stretchiness and elasticity.

Endovenous laser ablation: A procedure that uses laser energy to close varicose veins without scarring.

Epidermis: The thinnest, outer layer of the skin, which provides protection from the environment. The epidermis is made up of five layers: stratum germinativum, stratum spinosum, stratum granulosum, stratum lucidum and stratum corneum.

Exfoliate: To remove the outer skin layer consisting of dead cells.

Eye lift: See "blepharoplasty"

Facelift: See "rhytidectomy"

Fascia: A type of connective tissue that forms the lining of muscles.

Fractional laser resurfacing: A procedure that removes the outer surface of the skin in a scattered fashion. It reduces wrinkles and brown spots.

Freckle: A brown spot that appears on the skin as a result of sun exposure.

Hyperpigmentation: A condition seen as dark spots on the skin.

Hypertrophic scar: A thickened, raised scar.

Hypopigmentation: A condition in which there is lightening of the skin, representing an absence or decrease in skin pigment.

JUVEDERM®: A dermal filler made from hyaluronic acid gel used to fill wrinkles and replace volume.

Keloid scar: A type of scar that grows beyond the site of an injury. Caused by the formation of excess collagen. This condition has a genetic basis.

Keratin: Keratin is a protein that forms the rigidity of your skin, hair, and nails.

L-ascorbic acid: L-ascorbic acid is a form of Vitamin C.

Laser liposuction: A surgical procedure that reduces fat with laser energy followed by liposuction. Sometimes referred to as CoolLipo or SmartLipo.

Lentigines: See "age spots"

Lidocaine: An anesthetic often delivered in the form of an injection, similar to what is used by dentists to numb the teeth.

Lifestyle Lift: A national business franchise that performs 1-hour mini-facelifts.

Lip Augmentation: A procedure that increases lip volume or improves shape. Often done via injectable fillers.

Lipectomy: See "liposuction"

Lipoplasty: See "liposuction"

Liposuction: A cosmetic procedure that removes fat from

the body, often using suction and small tubes called cannulas.

Mammoplasty: A procedure that changes the size and/or shape of the breast. See "breast augmentation"

Mastectomy: The surgical removal of the breast, in part or in total.

Mastopexy: A surgical procedure, also called breast lift, which lifts the breast to a higher position, often combined with breast augmentation.

Melanocytes: The skin cells that produce pigment.

Melanoma: The most dangerous form of skin cancer that can be fatal if left untreated.

Mesotherapy: Treatments consisting of the injection of medicines, vitamins, or amino acids under the skin. Often used to reduce areas of fat or cellulite. Also termed lipo-dissolve.

Melasma: A condition in which brown patches of skin pigment are seen on the face, often on the cheeks and brow. This occurs in half of all women during pregnancy

Oculoplastics: Also called oculofacial plastics, this refers to the field of plastic surgery related to the eyelids, eyebrows, orbital bones, and the face.

Pectoralis: The largest muscle of the chest. Breast implants may be placed above or below this muscle.

Perlane: A dermal filler made from hyaluronic acid gel used to fill wrinkles and replace volume. Results last from 6-12 months.

Photoaging: The skin changes that occur with prolonged sun exposure, including deep and fine lines and age spots.

Platysma: The sheet-like muscle found under the skin of the neck that is responsible for vertical neck bands referred to as many as a "turkey waddle".

Platysmaplasty: A surgical procedure that improves the contour of the neck by tightening the platysma muscle. Often performed as part of a neck lift.

Ptosis: The drooping of a body part, most commonly referring to the eyelids or breasts.

Radiesse: A dermal filler with the consistency of bone paste consisting of hydroxylapatite that fills wrinkles and replaces volume. Results last from 9-18 months.

Restylane: A dermal filler made from hyaluronic acid gel used to fill wrinkles and replace volume. Results last from 4-6 months.

Retinol: A derivative of Vitamin A found in many skin care creams that reduces the development of wrinkles and increases skin growth.

Rhinoplasty: A cosmetic procedure also called nose job that improves the appearance of the nose.

Rhytidectomy: A surgical procedure also termed face lift which tightens the lower face muscles and skin, reducing jowls and neck looseness.

Rosacea: An inflammatory skin condition seen as redness on the face, including the cheeks and nose.

Sebaceous glands: The skin structures that produce oil.

Sclerotherapy: A medical procedure that eliminates varicose veins and "spider veins" with the injection of a liquid or foam solution.

Sculptra: A dermal filler consisting of poly-L-lactic acid that replaces facial volume, lasting for years.

Spider vein: A small, thread-like vein that can be seen through the surface of the skin.

Subcutaneous: A term referring to the area below the skin, where fat often resides.

Sun protection factor: Also described as "SPF", the sun protection factor is the amount of the protection a sunscreen provides. The higher the SPF, the greater the protection.

Suture: The stitches used to close an incision.

Thread lift: A method of lifting droopy neck and jowls with barbed stitches. This method has lost popularity because the results do not last for more than 1 year.

Tumescent: A form of anesthetic frequently used in liposuction and other cosmetic procedures. It consists of a fluid often containing dilute lidocaine and epinephrine.

Varicose vein: Enlarged, twisted veins found under the skin surface.

VelaShape: A device that delivers radiofrequency energy and infrared light, designed to reduce areas of cellulite.

6396500R0

Made in the USA
Charleston, SC
19 October 2010